Health Systems in Transition

Second Edition

Gregory P. Marchildon, *University of Regina, Canada*

UNIVERSITY OF TORONTO PRESS
Toronto Buffalo London

Canada:

Health System Review 2013

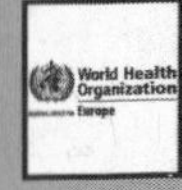

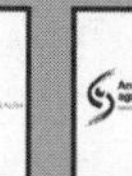
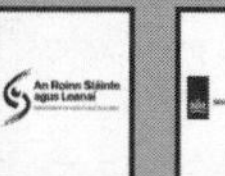
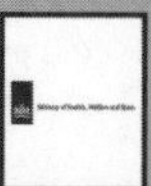

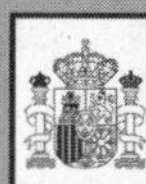

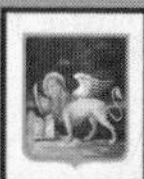
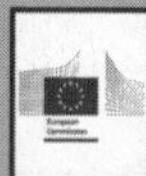
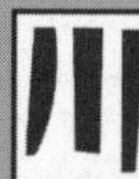
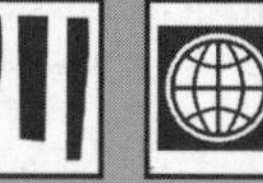
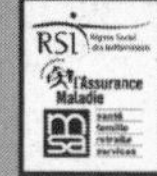
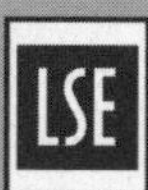
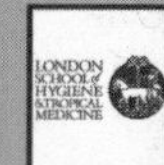

The European Observatory on Health Systems and Policies is a partnership between the WHO Regional Office for Europe, the Governments of Belgium, Finland, Ireland, the Netherlands, Norway, Slovenia, Spain, Sweden and the Veneto Region of Italy, the European Commission, the European Investment Bank, the World Bank, UNCAM (French National Union of Health Insurance Funds), the London School of Economics and Political Science, and the London School of Hygiene & Tropical Medicine.

Published by the WHO Regional Office for Europe on behalf of the European Observatory on Health Systems and Policies under the title Health Systems in Transition: Canada

Published in North America by University of Toronto Press, 2013
Toronto Buffalo London
www.utppublishing.com
Printed in Canada

ISBN 978-0-8020-9721-7

Printed on acid-free, 100% post-consumer recycled paper with vegetable-based inks.

Publication cataloguing information is available from Library and Archives Canada.

University of Toronto Press acknowledges the financial assistance to its publishing program of the Canada Council for the Arts and the Ontario Arts Council.

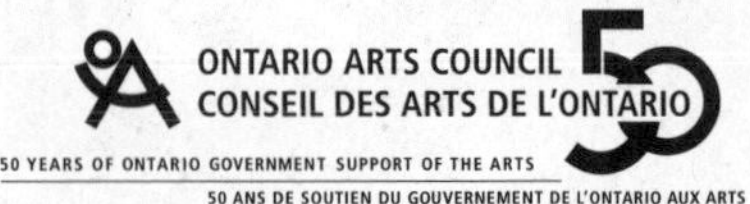

University of Toronto Press acknowledges the financial support of the Government of Canada through the Canada Book Fund for its publishing activities.

Contents

Preface

The Health Systems in Transition (HiT) series consists of country-based reviews that provide a detailed description of a health system and of reform and policy initiatives in progress or under development in a specific country. Each review is produced by country experts in collaboration with the Observatory's staff. In order to facilitate comparisons between countries, reviews are based on a template, which is revised periodically. The template provides detailed guidelines and specific questions, definitions and examples needed to compile a report.

HiTs seek to provide relevant information to support policy-makers and analysts in the development of health systems in Europe. They are building blocks that can be used:

- to learn in detail about different approaches to the organization, financing and delivery of health services and the role of the main actors in health systems;
- to describe the institutional framework, the process, content and implementation of health care reform programmes;
- to highlight challenges and areas that require more in-depth analysis;
- to provide a tool for the dissemination of information on health systems and the exchange of experiences of reform strategies between policy-makers and analysts in different countries; and
- to assist other researchers in more in-depth comparative health policy analysis.

Compiling the reviews poses a number of methodological problems. In many countries, there is relatively little information available on the health system and the impact of reforms. Due to the lack of a uniform data source, quantitative data on health services are based on a number of different sources, including the World Health Organization (WHO) Regional Office for Europe's European Health for All database, data from national statistical offices, Eurostat, the Organisation for Economic Co-operation and Development (OECD) Health Data, data from the International Monetary Fund (IMF), the World Bank's World Development Indicators and any other relevant sources considered useful by the authors. Data collection methods and definitions sometimes vary, but typically are consistent within each separate review.

There have been some challenges in adapting the HiT template to the Canadian case due largely to the inability to exploit WHO European data and the difficulty of applying terminology rooted in European history and health reform experience to Canada. Since the WHO European Health for All database does not include Canadian data, it was necessary to compare Canada using OECD and other data sources. For most of these comparisons, Canada was compared with a smaller set of countries than is customary in HiTs. Five countries were selected for systematic quantitative comparisons with Canada based on historical, political, economic and health policy criteria: Australia, France, Sweden, the United Kingdom and the United States. To avoid confusion with an identically named federal programme in the United States, medicare in Canada is spelled without a capital "M".

Comments and suggestions for the further development and improvement of the HiT series are most welcome and can be sent to info@obs.euro.who.int.

HiTs and HiT summaries are available on the Observatory's web site at http://www.healthobservatory.eu.

Acknowledgements

The HiT on Canada was produced by the European Observatory on Health Systems and Policies.

This edition was written by Gregory P. Marchildon (University of Regina). It was edited by Anna Sagan, Research Fellow, working with the support of Sarah Thomson, Research Director, both from the Observatory's team at the London School of Economics and Political Science. Sara Allin (University of Toronto and Canadian Institute for Health Information) contributed to the report by reviewing part of an earlier draft. The basis for this edition was the previous HiT on Canada, which was published in 2005, written by Gregory Marchildon and edited by Sara Allin.

The Observatory and the authors are grateful to Geoffrey Ballinger (Canadian Institute for Health Information), Jeremiah Hurley (McMaster University), Arthur Sweetman (McMaster University) and Carolyn Tuohy (University of Toronto) for reviewing the report.

Special thanks go also to the various (anonymous) employees of Health Canada and the Public Health Agency of Canada for their assistance in providing information and for their invaluable comments on previous drafts of the manuscript and suggestions about plans and current policy options in the Canadian health system. In addition, the author has benefited from the research assistance provided by his graduate students including Adam Mills, Michael Sherar, Kim Hill, Cassandra Opikokew and Colleen Walsh.

Thanks are also extended to the WHO Regional Office for Europe for their European Health for All database from which data on health services were extracted; to the OECD for the data on health services in western Europe; and to the World Bank for the data on health expenditure in central and eastern European countries. Thanks are also due to national institutions that have provided statistical data and particularly to the Canada Institute for Health

Information (CIHI), the Public Health Agency of Canada (PHAC) and Statistic Canada. The HiT reflects data available in January 2012, unless otherwise indicated.

The European Observatory is a partnership between the WHO Regional Office for Europe, the Governments of Belgium, Finland, Ireland, the Netherlands, Norway, Slovenia, Spain, Sweden and the Veneto Region of Italy, the European Commission, the European Investment Bank, the World Bank, UNCAM (French National Union of Health Insurance Funds), the London School of Economics and Political Science and the London School of Hygiene & Tropical Medicine. The Observatory team working on the HiT profiles is led by Josep Figueras, Director, and Elias Mossialos, Co-Director, and the heads of the research hubs, Martin McKee, Reinhard Busse and Richard Saltman. The production and copy-editing process was coordinated by Jonathan North, with the support of Pat Hinsley. Administrative and production support for preparing the HiT was provided by Caroline White. Additional support came from Mary Allen (copy-editing), Steve Still (design and layout) and Jane Ward (proofreading).

List of abbreviations

Abbreviations	
AB	Alberta (province)
ACHDHR	Advisory Committee on Health Delivery and Human Resources (F/P/T)
ALOS	Average length of stay
BC	British Columbia (province)
CADTH	Canadian Agency for Drugs and Technologies in Health
CAM	complementary and alternative medicine
CBS	Canadian Blood Services
CCHS	Canadian Community Health Survey
CDR	Common Drug Review (administered by CADTH)
CFNU	Canadian Federation of Nurses Unions
CHA	Canada Health Act
CHMS	Canadian Health Measures Survey
CHST	Canadian Health and Social Transfer
CIHI	Canadian Institute for Health Information
CIHR	Canadian Institutes of Health Research
CMA	Canadian Medical Association
CNA	Canadian Nurses Association
CT	computed tomography
CPHA	Canadian Public Health Association
DTCA	Direct-to-consumer advertising
ED	Emergency department
EHR	electronic health record
EPF	Established Programs Financing
FFS	Fee-for-service
F/P/T	federal–provincial–territorial
GATS	*General Agreement on Trade in Services*
GDP	gross domestic product
HCC	Health Council of Canada
HDI	Human Development Index

Abbreviations	
HHR	Health Human resource
HPRAC	Health Professionals Regulatory Advisory Council
HTA	health technology assessment
ICT	information and communications technology
IDI	International Telecommunication Union Development Index
IMG	International Medical graduates
IT	Information technology
LHIN	Local Health Integration Networks
MB	Manitoba (province)
MCHP	Manitoba Centre for Health Policy
MRI	magnetic resonance imaging
NAFTA	North American Free Trade Agreement
NB	New Brunswick (province)
NL	Newfoundland and Labrador (province)
NS	Nova Scotia (province)
NU	Nunavut (territory)
NWT	Northwest Territories (territory)
OECD	Organisation for Economic Co-operation and Development
ON	Ontario (province)
OOP	out of pocket
PEI	Prince Edward Island (province)
PHAC	Public Health Agency of Canada
PHI	private health insurance
PMPRB	Patented Medicine Prices Review Board
P/T	Provincial and Territorial
QC	Quebec (province)
RCMP	Royal Canadian Mounted Police
RCPSC	Royal College of Physicians and Surgeons of Canada
RHA	regional health authority
RN	registered nurse
RNAO	Registered Nurses Association of Ontario
SK	Saskatchewan (province)
THE	Total health expenditure
WCB	Workers' Compensation Board
WHO	World Health Organization
YK	Yukon (territory)

List of tables and figures

Tables

Tables

Figures

Abstract

Canada is a high-income country with a population of 33 million people. Its economic performance has been solid despite the recession that began in 2008. Life expectancy in Canada continues to rise and is high compared with most OECD countries; however, infant and maternal mortality rates tend to be worse than in countries such as Australia, France and Sweden. About 70% of total health expenditure comes from the general tax revenues of the federal, provincial and territorial governments. Most public revenues for health are used to provide universal medicare (medically necessary hospital and physician services that are free at the point of service for residents) and to subsidise the costs of outpatient prescription drugs and long-term care. Health care costs continue to grow at a faster rate than the economy and government revenue, largely driven by spending on prescription drugs. In the last five years, however, growth rates in pharmaceutical spending have been matched by hospital spending and overtaken by physician spending, mainly due to increased provider remuneration.

The governance, organization and delivery of health services is highly decentralized, with the provinces and territories responsible for administering medicare and planning health services. In the last ten years there have been no major pan-Canadian health reform initiatives but individual provinces and territories have focused on reorganizing or fine tuning their regional health systems and improving the quality, timeliness and patient experience of primary, acute and chronic care. The medicare system has been effective in providing Canadians with financial protection against hospital and physician costs. However, the narrow scope of services covered under medicare has produced important gaps in coverage and equitable access may be a challenge in these areas.

Executive summary

Introduction

The second largest country in the world as measured by area, Canada is a high-income country with an advanced industrial economy. Since 2006, Canada's economic performance has been relatively solid despite the recession that began in 2008. Although revenue growth has remained robust, the federal government as well as a number of provincial governments have also reduced tax rates in recent years. At the same time, health care costs continue to grow at rates that exceed economic and government revenue growth, raising concerns about the fiscal sustainability of health expenditure financed through the public sector.

Canada is a constitutional monarchy based on a British-style parliamentary system. It is also a federation with two constitutionally recognized orders of government. The first order is the central or "federal" government, which is responsible for certain aspects of health and pharmaceutical regulation and safety, as well as the financing and administration of health benefits and services for specific populations. The second, but constitutionally equal, order of government consists of the ten provincial governments, which bear the principal responsibility for a broad range of social policy programmes and services including the bulk of publicly financed and administered health services.

Life expectancy in Canada has continued to increase since 1980, especially for males, and is relatively high compared with most OECD countries, even though infant mortality and maternal mortality rates tend to be worse than those in Australia, France and (especially) Sweden. The two main causes of death in Canada are cancer (malignant neoplasms) and cardiovascular disease, both of which have occupied the top positions since 2000.

Organization and governance

Canada has a predominantly publicly financed health system with approximately 70% of health expenditures financed through the general tax revenues of the federal, provincial and territorial (F/P/T) governments. At the same time, the governance, organization and delivery of health services is highly decentralized for at least three reasons: (1) provincial and territorial responsibility for the funding and delivery of most health care services; (2) the status of physicians as independent contractors; and (3) the existence of multiple organizations, from regional health authorities (RHAs) to privately governed hospitals, that operate at arm's length from provincial governments.

Saskatchewan was the first province to implement a universal hospital services plan in 1947. Ten years later, the federal government passed the Hospital Insurance and Diagnostic Services Act which outlined the common conditions that provincial governments had to satisfy in order to receive shared-cost financing through federal transfers. In 1962, Saskatchewan extended coverage to include physician services and, in 1966, the federal government introduced the Medical Care Act to cost-share single-payer insurance for physician costs with provincial governments. By 1971, all provinces had universal coverage for hospital and physician services. In 1984, the federal government replaced the two previous acts with the Canada Health Act, a law that set pan-Canadian standards for hospital, diagnostic and medical care services.

Most health system planning is conducted at the provincial and territorial levels although in some jurisdictions RHAs engage in more detailed planning of services for their defined populations. Some provincial ministries of health and RHAs are aided in their planning by provincial quality councils and specialized health technology assessment (HTA) agencies. In recent years, there has been a trend towards greater centralization in terms of reducing or eliminating RHAs. Most health professions self-regulate under legal frameworks established by provincial and territorial governments.

The federal government's activities range from funding and facilitating data gathering and research to regulating prescription drugs and public health while continuing to support the national dimensions of medicare through large funding transfers to the provinces and territories. The F/P/T governments collaborate through conferences, councils and working groups comprised of ministers and deputy ministers of health. In recent years, this has been supplemented by specialized intergovernmental bodies responsible for data collection and dissemination, HTA, patient safety, information and communications technology (ICT) and the management of blood products. Nongovernmental organizations at both federal and provincial levels influence policy direction and the management of public health care in Canada.

Financing

The public sector in Canada is responsible for roughly 70% of total health expenditure. After a period of spending restraint in the early to mid-1990s, government expenditures have grown rapidly, a rate of growth exceeded only by private health expenditure. Since health expenditure has grown more rapidly than the growth in either the economy or public revenues, this has triggered concerns about the fiscal sustainability of public health care. Contrary to popular perception, demographic ageing has not yet been a major cost driver of health system costs in Canada. Over the last two decades, prescription drugs have been a major cost driver, but in the last five years, the growth in this sector has been matched by hospital spending and overtaken by physician expenditures. In the case of physicians, a primary cost driver has been increased remuneration, and in the case of hospitals, it is a combination of more hiring and increased remuneration for existing staff.

Almost all revenues for public health spending come from the general tax revenues of F/P/T governments, a considerable portion of which are used to provide universal medicare – medically necessary hospital and physician services that are free at the point of service for residents in all provinces and territories. The remaining amount is used to subsidize other types of health care including long-term care and prescription drugs. While the provinces raise the majority of funds through own-source revenues, they also receive less than a quarter of their health financing from the Canada Health Transfer, an annual cash transfer from the federal government. The provinces and territories are responsible for administering their own tax-funded and universal hospital and medicare plans. Medically necessary hospital, diagnostic and physician services are free at the point of service for all provincial and territorial residents. Historically, the federal government played an important role in encouraging the introduction of these plans, discouraging the use of user fees and maintaining insurance portability among provinces and territories by tying contributory transfers to the upholding of these conditions. Beyond the universal basket of hospital and physician services, provincial and territorial governments subsidize or provide other health goods and services such as prescription drug coverage and long-term care (including home care). In contrast to hospital and physician services, these provincial programmes generally target sub populations on the basis of age or income and can require user fees. On the private side, out-of-pocket (OOP) payments and purchases of private health insurance (PHI) are responsible for most health revenues. The vast majority of PHI comes in the form of employment-based insurance for non-medicare goods and services, including prescription drugs, dental care and vision care. PHI does not compete with the provincial and territorial "single payer" systems for medicare.

Physical and human resources

The non-financial inputs into the Canadian health system include buildings, equipment, information technology (IT) and the health workforce. The ability of any health system to provide timely access to quality health services depends not only on the sufficiency of physical and human resources but on finding the appropriate balance among these resources. Both the sufficiency and the balance of resources need to be adjusted continually by F/P/T governments in response to the constantly evolving technology, health care practices and health needs of Canadians.

Between the mid-1970s and 2000, capital investment in hospitals declined. Small hospitals were closed in many parts of Canada and acute care services were consolidated. Despite recent reinvestments in hospital stock by provincial and territorial governments, in particular in medical equipment, imaging technologies and ICT, the number of acute care beds per capita has continued to fall, in part a result of the increase in day surgeries. While most of Canada's supply of advanced diagnostic technologies is roughly comparable to levels in other OECD countries, it scores poorly in terms of its effective use of ICT relative to other high-income countries. However, in recent years, some advances have been made in this area.

After a lengthy period in the 1990s when the supply of physicians and nurses, as well as other public health care workers, was reduced because of government cutbacks, the health workforce has grown since 2000. Private sector health professionals have seen even more substantial growth during this period. Medical and nursing faculties have expanded in order to produce more graduates. At the same time, there has been an increase in the immigration of foreign-educated doctors and nurses and lower emigration to other countries such as the United States.

Provision of services

Although it is difficult to generalize given the decentralized nature of health services administration and delivery in Canada, the typical patient pathway starts with a visit to a family physician, who then determines the course of basic treatment, if any. In most provinces, family physicians act as gatekeepers: they decide whether their patients should obtain diagnostic tests, prescription drugs or be referred to medical specialists. However, provincial ministries of health have renewed efforts to reform primary care in the last decade. Many of these reform efforts focus on moving from the traditional physician-only practice to interprofessional primary care teams that provide a broader range of primary health care services on a 24-hour, 7-day-a-week basis (although progress here is slow). In cases where the patient does not have a regular family physician or needs help after regular clinic hours, the first point of contact may be a walk-in medical clinic or a hospital emergency department.

Illness prevention services, including disease screening, may be provided by a family physician, a public health office or a dedicated screening programme. All provincial and territorial governments have public health and health promotion initiatives. They also conduct health surveillance and manage epidemic response. While the Public Health Agency of Canada (PHAC) develops and manages programmes supporting public health throughout Canada, the responsibility for most day-to-day public health activities and supporting infrastructure remains with the provincial and territorial governments.

Almost all acute care is provided in public or non-profit-making private hospitals although some specialized ambulatory and advanced diagnostic services may be provided in private profit-making clinics. Most hospitals have an emergency department that is fed by independent emergency medical service units providing first response care to patients while being transported to emergency departments.

As for prescription drugs, every provincial and territorial government has a prescription drug plan that covers outpatient prescription drugs for designated populations (e.g. seniors and social assistance recipients), with the federal government providing drug coverage for eligible First Nations and Inuit users. These public insurers depend heavily on HTA, including the Common Drug Review (CDR) conducted by the Canadian Agency for Drugs and Technologies in Health (CADTH), to determine which drugs should be included in their respective formularies. Despite the creation of a National Pharmaceuticals

Strategy following the *10-Year Plan* agreed to by first ministers in 2004, there has been little progress on a pan-Canadian catastrophic drug coverage programme.

Rehabilitation and long-term care policies and services, including home and community care, palliative care and support for informal carers, vary considerably among provinces and territories. Until the 1960s, the locus of most mental health care was in large, provincially run psychiatric hospitals. Since deinstitutionalization, individuals with mental illnesses are diagnosed and treated by psychiatrists on an outpatient basis even though they may spend periods of time in the psychiatric wards of hospitals. Family physicians provide the majority of primary mental health care.

Unlike long-term care and mental health, almost all dental care is privately funded in Canada. As a consequence of access being largely based on income, outcomes are highly inequitable. Complementary and alternative medicine (CAM) is, with a few exceptions (e.g. chiropractors in some provinces) also privately funded and delivered.

Due to the disparities in health outcomes for Aboriginal peoples, as well as the historical challenge of servicing some of the most remote communities in Canada, F/P/T governments have established a number of targeted programmes and services. While Aboriginal health status has improved in the postwar period, a large gap in health status continues to separate the Aboriginal population from most other Canadians.

Principal health reforms

Since 2005, when the first edition of this study was published, there have been no major pan-Canadian health reform initiatives. However, individual provincial and territorial ministries of health have concentrated on two categories of reform, one involving the reorganization or fine tuning of their regional health systems, and the second linked to improving the quality, timeliness and patient experience of primary, acute and chronic care.

The main purpose of regionalization (i.e. the introduction of RHAs to manage services as purchasers or purchaser–providers) was to gain the benefits of vertical integration by managing facilities and providers across a broad continuum of health services, in particular to improve the coordination of "downstream" curative services with more "upstream" public health and illness prevention services and interventions. In the last ten years, in an attempt to capture economies of scale and scope in service delivery as well as reduce infrastructure costs, there has been a trend to greater centralization, with provincial ministries of health reducing the number of RHAs. Two provinces, Alberta and Prince Edward Island, now have a single RHA responsible for coordinating all acute and long-term care services (but not primary care) in their respective areas.

Influenced chiefly by quality improvement initiatives in the United States and the United Kingdom, provincial ministries of health have established institutions and mechanisms to improve the quality, safety, timeliness and responsiveness of health services. Six provinces have established health quality councils to accelerate quality improvement initiatives. Two provincial governments also launched patient-centred initiatives aimed at improving the experience of both patients and caregivers. Most ministries and RHAs also implemented some aspects of performance measurement in an effort to improve outcomes and processes. Patient dissatisfaction with long wait times in hospital emergency departments and for certain types of elective surgery such as joint replacements has triggered efforts in all provinces to better manage and reduce waiting times.

In contrast, there has been more limited progress on the intergovernmental front since the first ministers' *10-Year Plan to Strengthen Health Care* in 2004. Following that meeting, provincial and territorial governments used additional federal cash transfers to invest in shortening waiting times in priority areas, reinvigorating primary care reform and providing additional coverage for home care services that could substitute for hospital care. While a number of provincial and territorial governments introduced some form of catastrophic drug coverage for certain groups of their own residents, they achieved very little in forging a pan-Canadian approach to prescription drug coverage and management.

Assessment of the health system

In assessing performance, the medicare system has been effective in financially protecting Canadians against high-cost hospital and medical care. At the same time, the narrow scope of universal services covered under medicare has produced important gaps in coverage. In the cases of prescription drugs and dental care, for example, depending on employment and province or territory of residence, these gaps are filled by PHI and, at least in the case of drug therapies, by provincial plans that target seniors and the very poor. Where public coverage does not fill in the cracks left by PHI, equitable access is a major challenge. Since the majority of funding for health care comes from general tax revenues of the F/P/T governments, and the revenue sources range from progressive to proportionate, there is equity in financing. However, to the extent that financing is OOP and through employment-based insurance benefits that are associated with better-paid jobs, there is less equity in financing overall.

There are disparities in terms of access to health care but outside of a few areas such as dental care and mental health care, they do not appear to be large. For example, there appears to be a pro-poor bias in terms of primary care use but a pro-rich bias in the use of specialist physician services, but the gap in both cases is not large. There is an east–west economic gradient, with differences between less wealthy provinces in eastern Canada and more wealthy provinces in western Canada. This is systematically addressed through equalization payments from federal revenue sources made to "have-not" provinces to ensure that they have the revenues necessary to provide comparable levels of public services, including health care, without resorting to prohibitively high tax rates.

While Canadians are generally satisfied with the financial protection offered by medicare, they are less satisfied with access to health care. In particular, starting in the 1990s, they became dissatisfied with access to physicians and crowded emergency departments in hospitals, as well as lengthening waiting times for non-urgent surgery. Based on the results of a 2010 survey of patients by the Commonwealth Fund, for example, Canada ranked behind Australia, France, Sweden, the United Kingdom and the United States in terms of patient experience with waiting times for physician care and non-urgent surgery. Using more objective indicators of health system performance such as amenable mortality, however, assessment of Canadian health system performance is more positive, with much better outcomes than those observed in the United Kingdom and the United States, although not as good as Australia, Sweden and France. Canadian performance on an index of health care quality indicators has also improved over the past decade as provincial governments, assisted by health quality councils and other organizations, more systemically implement quality improvement measures. Finally, governments, health care organizations and providers are making more efforts to improve the overall patient experience.

1. Introduction

The second largest country in the world as measured by area, Canada is a high-income country with an advanced industrial economy. Since 2006, Canada's economic performance has been relatively solid despite the recession that began in 2008. Although revenue growth has remained robust, the federal government as well as a number of provincial governments have also reduced tax rates in recent years. At the same time, health care costs continue to rise at rates that exceed economic and government revenue growth, raising continuing concerns about the fiscal sustainability of health expenditures, financing through the public sector.

In terms of the form of government, Canada is a constitutional monarchy based on a British-style parliamentary system. It is also a federation with two constitutionally recognized orders of government. The first order is the central or "federal" government. The second but constitutionally equal order of government consists of the ten provincial governments in Canada, which bear the principal responsibility for a broad range of social policy programmes and services including the bulk of publicly financed and administered health services.

Life expectancy in Canada has continued to increase since 1980, especially for males, and is relatively high compared with most OECD countries, even though infant mortality and maternal mortality rates tend to be worse than those in Australia, France and (especially) Sweden. The two main causes of death in Canada are cancer (malignant neoplasms) and cardiovascular disease, both of which have occupied the top positions since 2000.

1.1 Geography and sociodemography

Canada is a large country with a land mass of 9 093 507 km^2 (or 9 984 670 km^2 including inland water). The mainland spans a distance of 5514 km from east to west, and 4634 km from north to south. The country is bounded by the United States to the south and the north-west (Alaska), the Pacific Ocean in the west, the Atlantic Ocean in the east, and the Arctic Ocean in the far north. The terrain of the country ranges from extensive mountain ranges to large continental plains, from huge inland lakes and boreal forests to the vast tundra of the Arctic. The climate is northern in nature with a long and cold winter season experienced in almost all parts of the country (Fig. 1.1).

Fig. 1.1
Map of Canada

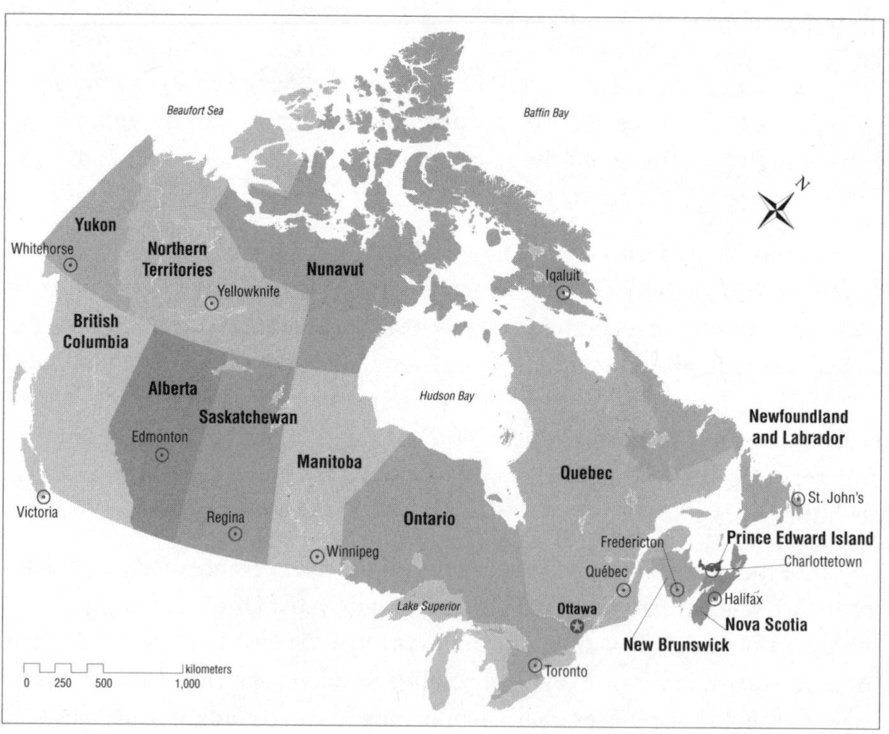

Source: Author's own compilation.

The United States, a country with almost 10 times the population of Canada and a higher level of per capita income, exerts considerable cultural and economic influence on the daily life of Canadians. Although there are major, even fundamental, differences in how public health care is funded and organized in the two countries, domestic debates concerning access and quality as well as health system reform are highly influenced by Canadian perceptions of the state of health care in the United States.

Although it has a large land mass, Canada's population was less than 34 million in 2011. The two largest cities are Toronto and Montreal, with 5.7 million and 3.9 million inhabitants, respectively, living in the cities and surrounding areas, defined as census metropolitan areas.[1] In contrast, the country's capital city, Ottawa, has a census metropolitan area population of 1.2 million. Although Canada has one of the lowest human population densities in the world (3.4 persons per km^2), most of the population is concentrated in southern urban centres that are close to the United States border. A relatively small number of Canadians lives in the immense rural and more northerly regions of the country. Most new immigrants live in Canada's largest cities while the majority of the country's Aboriginal (First Nation, Inuit and Métis) citizens live on rural reserves, land claim regions in the Arctic or in the poorer city neighbourhoods.

Table 1.1

Population in persons and percentages in all the Canadian provinces and territories (capital cities in parentheses), 2011

Province/territory	Number	% of total
British Columbia (Victoria)	4 400 057	13.14
Alberta (Edmonton)	3 645 257	10.89
Saskatchewan (Regina)	1 033 381	3.09
Manitoba (Winnipeg)	1 208 268	3.61
Ontario (Toronto)	12 851 821	38.39
Quebec (Québec)	7 903 001	23.61
New Brunswick (Fredericton)	751 171	2.24
Nova Scotia (Halifax)	921 727	2.75
Prince Edward Island (Charlottetown)	140 204	0.42
Newfoundland and Labrador (St. John's)	514 536	1.54
Yukon (Whitehorse)	33 897	0.10
Northwest Territories (Yellowknife)	41 462	0.12
Nunavut (Iqaluit)	31 906	0.10
Canada (Ottawa)	**33 476 688**	**100.00**

Source: Statistics Canada (2011).

1 According to Statistics Canada, a census metropolitan area has one or more neighbouring municipalities situated around a large urban core. For example, while there are 5.7 million people in the Toronto census metropolitan area, the population residing in the urban core of Toronto was estimated at 2.5 million in 2006, the last census year.

In terms of a health system serving populations in Canada, four factors should be considered: (1) demographic ageing; (2) rural and remote communities and populations; (3) cultural diversity resulting from high rates of immigration; and (4) unique rights and claims pertaining to Aboriginal peoples and their historic displacement and marginalization relative to the majority of Canadians. Each of these issues is summarized below.

Despite the demographic ageing of its population since 1970, Canada has a smaller proportion of older citizens than most countries in Western Europe. Moreover, Canada's age dependency ratio – defined as the ratio of children (1–14 years) and senior adults (≥65 years) to the working-age population – is also lower than in the five comparator countries (Table 1.2).

Table 1.2
Selected human development indicators for Canada and selected countries, 2011

Selected indicators	Canada	Australia	France	Sweden	United Kingdom	United States
Human Development Index global rank (actual index value)	6 (0.908)	2 (0.929)	20 (0.884)	10 (0.904)	28 (0.863)	4 (0.910)
Gross national income per capita (PPP US$)	35 166	34 431	30 462	35 837	33 296	43 017
Total expenditure on health, per capita (PPP US$), 2007	3 900	3 357	3 709	3 323	2 991	7 286
Age dependency ratio (ratio of population 0–14 and 65+ to population 15–64 years), per 100 people	44.5	50.7	54.9	54.2	50.1	52.0
Income Gini coefficient, 2000–2010 [a]	32.6	35.2	32.7	25.0	36.0	40.8
Mean years of schooling	12.1	12.0	10.6	11.7	9.3	12.4
Political voice (% of population who voiced opinion to public official) [a]	20	23	23	29	24	32
Gender inequality rank in the world	20	18	10	1	47	34
Adolescent fertility rate, 2011*, per 1000 women aged 15–19	14.0	16.5	7.2	6.0	29.6	41.2
Life expectancy at birth, years	81.0	81.9	81.5	81.4	80.2	78.5
Health-adjusted life expectancy, years	73	74	73	74	72	70
Overall life satisfaction, 2006–2009, scale of 0 (least) to 10 (most)	7.7	7.5	6.8	7.5	7.0	7.2

Sources: UNDP (2011) for income Gini coefficient, political voice and death rates; [a] UNDP (2010).
Note: * Annual average for 2010–2015 (UNDP, 2011).

Senior adults made up 14% of the population in 2009 compared to 9% in 1980, but they are projected to constitute 23% of the population by 2030 (Statistics Canada, 2009). The decrease in family size over time has served to cushion the age dependency ratio, with the birth rate declining from 15 per 1000 population in 1980 to 11 per 1000 population in 2005 (Table 1.3).

Table 1.3
Population indicators, 1980–2010 (selected years)

	1980	1990	1995	2000	2005	2010
Total population (millions)	24.6	27.8	29.4	30.8	32.3	34.1
Population, female (% of total)	50	50	51	50	50	50.4
Population aged 0–14 (% of total)	23	21	20	19	18	16.4
Population aged 65 and above (% of total)	9	11	12	13	13	14.1
Male population aged 80 and above (% of total)	1	2	2	2	2	3.0
Female population aged 80 and above (% of total)	2	3	3	4	4	4.0
Population growth (average annual growth rate)	1.3	1.5	0.8	0.9	1.0	1.1
Population density (people per sq km)	3	3	3	3	4	3.8
Fertility rate, total (births per woman)	2	2	2	1	2	1.7[a]
Birth rate, crude (per 1 000 people)	15	15	13	11	11	11.2[a]
Death rate, crude (per 1 000 people)	7	7	7	7	7	7.4[a]
Age dependency ratio (ratio of population 0–14 and 65+ to population 15–64 years), per 100 people	47	47	48	46	44	44.0
Rural population as % of total population	24	23	22	21	20	19.4

Sources: Statistics Canada (2011); World Bank (2011).
Note: [a] 2009 data.

Although the proportion of the population defined as rural has been steadily falling since 1980, rural populations are very unevenly distributed among Canadian provinces and territories. More than half the residents in Saskatchewan, New Brunswick, Nova Scotia, Prince Edward, Newfoundland and Labrador and the three territories live in rural regions far from metropolitan centres.[2]

As for population make-up, almost 20% of Canadian residents were born outside the country. The 2006 census reported more than 200 different ethnic origins and an estimated 41% of the population reported multiple ethnic ancestries (Statistics Canada, 2008). Table 1.4 provides the number and percentage of respondents in the census who reported single or multiple ethnic ancestries. While the majority of Canadians have British, French or other European ancestry, most recent immigrants come from outside Europe and have neither English nor French as their first language. They are clustered in Canada's largest cities, putting pressure on health care facilities in large urban centres to provide services in ways that can overcome cultural and linguistic barriers to access.

[2] These are classified as "rural non-metro-adjacent regions" and "rural northern and remote regions" by Statistics Canada.

Table 1.4
Ethnic self-identification of Canadian population, total population and percentage, 2006

Origin	Total population	Percentage (%)
British	11 098 610	35.5
Canadian	10 066 290	32.2
European	9 919 790	31.8
French	5 000 350	16.0
East and Southeast Asian	2 212 340	7.1
Aboriginal	1 678 235	5.4
South Asian	1 316 770	4.2
Other[a]	2 191 750	7.0

Source: Statistics Canada (2006).
Notes: Percentages are calculated as a proportion of the total number of 2006 census respondents. The sum exceeds 100% due to multiple ethnic origin responses. [a] Other includes African; Arab; West Asian; Latin, Central and South American; and from Oceania.

Canada also has an Aboriginal population made up of three distinct groupings: First Nations (North American Indians), Inuit and Métis. The terms "status Indians" and "registered Indians" are legal terms used by the Government of Canada to describe First Nations who are officially registered under the terms of the Indian Act and, therefore, qualify for specified entitlements and benefits, including "non-insured health benefits" financed and administered by the federal government. Registered Indians can live on or off reserves, many of which are located in rural and remote areas of Canada. Most Inuit live in the Arctic regions of Canada, mainly in settlements located on the shore of the Arctic Ocean. The Métis, the majority of whom are the descendants of Euro-Canadian and Aboriginal fur traders, are concentrated in Western Canada.

First Nations and Métis are affected disproportionately more by chronic diseases and conditions such as diabetes, hypertension, heart disease, tuberculosis, HIV and fetal alcohol spectrum disorder. First Nations people living on reserves also experience physical injuries at a much higher rate than the Canadian average. For example, Martens et al. (2002) found that injury hospitalization rates among First Nations peoples living in Manitoba were 3.7 times higher than those of all other provincial residents. Although Inuit populations are less affected by some diseases and conditions such as diabetes, heart disease and fetal alcohol spectrum disorder, due in part to more traditional and less sedentary lives, current trends in lifestyle and diet are likely to produce similarly poor health status outcomes in the future (Sharma et al., 2010). As a result of poorer health status, Aboriginal Canadians account for higher average utilization and cost of health care services than other Canadians.

1.2 Economic context

Canada is an advanced industrial economy with a substantial natural resource base. Measured in terms of per capita wealth, the country ranks among the richest nations in the world. In terms of income inequality as measured by the Gini coefficient, disposable incomes in Canada are more equal than in the United States, the United Kingdom and Australia but less equal than in Sweden and its Nordic neighbours, and the same as in France (UNDP, 2010). On the overall Human Development Index calculated by the United Nations Development Programme (UNDP, 2011), Canada ranked slightly below Australia (second) and the United States (fourth), but above Sweden, France and the United Kingdom in 2010 (see Table 1.2).

During the last five years, Canada's economic performance has been among the strongest in the OECD. Similar to Australia, Canada suffered less than most Western European nations and the United States from the global recession that began in 2008. Moreover, as a major exporter of resources, including oil and gas as well as foodstuffs, the country has benefited from the recent spike upwards in global commodity prices. As a result, the Canadian dollar (like the Australian dollar) has appreciated against both the United States dollar and the euro since the recession beginning in 2008. In the years following, unemployment rates in the country are also lower than those in the United States, the United Kingdom, France and Sweden (Table 1.5).

Despite this positive economic performance, health care costs continue to grow at rates that exceed government revenue growth, raising concerns about the future fiscal sustainability of public health care (OECD, 2010b). However, this is partly due to systematic tax cutting by federal and provincial governments. As a consequence, the ratio of federal tax revenues to gross domestic product (GDP), for example, declined from 14.6% in 1997–1998 to 13.7% by 2006–2007 (Ruggeri & Watson, 2008).

Table 1.5
Macroeconomic indicators, 1980–2009 (selected years)

	1980	1990	1995	2000	2005	2009
GDP, PPP (current international US$, billions)	271.3	541.9	666.2	874.1	1 132.0	1 329.9
GDP per capita, PPP (current international US$, thousands)	11.0	19.5	22.7	28.4	35.0	39.0
GDP average annual growth rate for the last 10 years (%), PPP (current international US$)	2.2	0.2	2.8	5.2	3.0	3.2
Public expenditure (% of GDP)	21.3	22.3	21.3	18.6	18.9	21.8
Cash surplus/deficit (% of GDP)	–	-4.9[a]	-4.0	2.2	1.3	-1.8[c]
Tax burden (% of GDP)	–	15.3[a]	13.7	15.3	13.8	11.8[c]
Central government debt (% of GDP)	–	–	–	–	44.0[b]	53.1[c]
Value added in industry (% of GDP)	36.9	31.3	30.7	33.2	32.4	31.5[d]
Value added in agriculture (% of GDP)	4.3	2.9	2.9	2.3	1.8	1.7[d]
Value added in services (% of GDP)	58.8	65.8	66.4	64.5	65.8	66.8[d]
Labour force (total in millions)	12.1	14.7	15.1	16.3	17.8	19.1[c]
Unemployment total (% of labour force)	7.5	8.1	9.5	6.8	6.8	8.3[c]
Income inequality (after-tax Gini coefficient)	35.3	35.7	36.3	39.2	39.3	39.4[c]
Real interest rate	3.8	10.6	6.2	3.0	1.1	-0.3
Official exchange rate (US$)	1.2	1.2	1.4	1.5	1.2	1.0

Sources: World Bank (2011); Statistics Canada (2012).
Notes: [a] 1991 data; [b] 2006 data; [c] 2009 data; [d] 2007 data.

1.3 Political context

Canada has two constitutionally recognized orders of government, the central or "federal" government and 10 provinces. While they do not enjoy the constitutional status of the provinces, the three northern territories exercise many of the same policy and programme responsibilities, including those for health care.

As measured by a number of criteria, including provincial control of revenues and expenditure relative to the central government, the country has become a more decentralized federation since the early 1960s (Watts, 2008). This trend has, in part, been driven by the struggle of successive administrations in Quebec seeking greater autonomy for their province from the federal government (Requejo, 2010). In recent years, other provincial governments have joined Quebec in demanding some redress of what they perceive as a fiscal imbalance between the ever-growing spending responsibilities of the provinces, especially for health care, relative to the much greater revenue-generating capacity of the central government. Some provincial governments (e.g. Alberta) have occasionally demanded less federal conditionality and greater flexibility in terms of the Canada Health Act.

Unlike the provinces and territories, local or municipal governments are not constitutionally recognized. Instead, they are political units created under provincial government law. Municipal and county governments are delegated authority and responsibility by the provinces for the delivery of local public services and infrastructure. Historically, local governments played a role, albeit modest, in the administration and delivery of health services. However, the Saskatchewan model of single-payer hospital and medical care services with a centralized payment system administered by provincial governments was eventually adopted by other provinces and territories (Taylor, 1987; Tuohy 2009).

Elections take place on average every four years for the federal House of Commons as well as for provincial and territorial legislatures under a "first-past-the-post" electoral system[3] based on F/P/T constituencies. Political competition occurs largely with the context of competitive and adversarial political parties.[4] Except for the social democratic New Democratic Party (NDP), provincial parties are organizationally separate from political parties at the federal level. The Prime Minister is the leader of the majority party in the House of Commons and appoints the cabinet of ministers from among the elected members, a system that is replicated in the provinces and one territory – Yukon. Currently, there are four national political parties that attempt to run candidates in all constituencies in Canada: the Conservative Party of Canada, the NDP, the Liberal Party of Canada and the Green Party of Canada. There is also a regional party – the Bloc Québécois – but its influence was severely diminished after the 2011 federal election. Established in the early 1990s to advance Quebec's independence from the Canadian federation, the Bloc regularly defends what it defines as Quebec's interests in the Parliament of Canada, and supports a progressive decentralization of power and authority from the central government to the provinces. In the federal election of 2006, the Conservative Party of Canada under leader Stephen Harper defeated a Liberal Government that had been in power since 1993. The Harper Conservatives were defeated on a motion of non-confidence but won a second minority government in 2008 and a majority government in 2011 (Table 1.6).

[3] Each voter selects one candidate. All votes are counted and the candidate with the most votes in a defined geographical constituency is the winner irrespective of the votes garnered by the candidate's political party on a national, provincial or territorial basis.

[4] There are two exceptions to this rule: the territorial governments in Nunavut and the Northwest Territories are formed by individual members elected without party affiliations, and cabinet membership is decided by the votes of the members of the legislative assemblies.

Table 1.6
Results of federal elections of 14 October 2008 and 2 May 2011

Political party	2008		2011	
	Seats	Popular vote (%)	Seats	Popular vote (%)
Conservative	143	37.6	166	39.6
New Democratic Party	37	18.2	103	30.6
Liberal	77	26.2	34	18.9
Bloc Québécois	49	10.0	4	6.0
Green Party	0	6.8	1	3.9
Independent	2	0.7	0	0.4
Other	0	0.5	0	0.6

Sources: Elections Canada (2008, 2011).

Internationally, Canada is a founding member of the United Nations and, because of its long history as a self-governing colony within the British Empire, an influential member of the Commonwealth of Nations. Due to its status as both a French-speaking and English-speaking jurisdiction, Canada is also a member of the Organisation Internationale de la Francophonie, as are the provinces of Quebec and New Brunswick.

Global health forms part of Canadian foreign policy and international development assistance. Canada is signatory to several international treaties that recognize the right to health, the most important of which are the Universal Declaration of Human Rights (1948) and the International Covenant on Economic, Social and Cultural Rights (1976). The Canadian Government played an important role in establishing the globally influential Ottawa Charter for Health Promotion in 1986, a declaration highlighting the impact of the social determinants of health, strongly influenced by the earlier Lalonde Report of 1974 (Kickbusch, 2003). In 1991, Canada ratified the United Nations Convention on the Rights of the Child and its provisions concerning the health and health care rights of children. In 1997, Canada became a member of the World Intellectual Property Organization Copyright Treaty, which has significant implications for prescription drug patenting as well as research and development in the medical sector generally.

Canada is also an active participant in the WHO and its regional office in the Americas – the Pan American Health Organization. Under the auspices of WHO, the Framework Convention on Tobacco Control (WHO, 2003) attempts to widen and strengthen public health measures to reduce tobacco consumption and thereby reduce its deleterious health consequences throughout the world. As a country that has succeeded in reducing its smoking rate dramatically over the past few decades, Canada has played a constructive role in the negotiation of this landmark convention and in facilitating a global effort to reduce tobacco consumption (Kapur, 2003; Roemer, Taylor & Lariviere, 2005). Canada was also a catalyst in the establishment of the 2001 Global Health Security Initiative (GHSI) led by the ministers or secretaries of health from eight countries (Canada, France, Germany, Italy, Japan, Mexico, the United Kingdom and the United States) and the European Commission with the WHO acting as a technical advisor. In addition to its work on strengthening global preparedness and response to threats of chemical, biological and radio-nuclear terrorism and the containment of contagious diseases, GHSI has developed a vaccine-procurement protocol. Canada has played a lead role with the WHO in identifying chronic disease prevention and control, and in helping establish a Framework Agreement for Cooperation on Chronic Diseases in 2005.

Additionally, Canada is a member of the World Trade Organization (WTO) and, with the United States and Mexico, a member of the North American Free Trade Agreement (NAFTA). NAFTA and the General Agreement on Trade in Services (GATS) under the WTO are very broad in their scope but both contain provisions that ostensibly protect public-sector health care services from coming under these trade rules. NAFTA, for example, exempts all "social services established or maintained for a public purpose" from its trade and investment liberalization provisions. In contrast, GATS only applies to those services or sectors that are explicitly made subject to the agreement, and countries such as Canada have chosen not to include its own public-sector health care services in GATS (Romanow, 2002; Ouellet, 2004). Nevertheless, there remains some anxiety about public sector health care being subject to trade laws, particularly hospital and medical services, fuelled by the apprehension that foreign corporations may eventually demand "national treatment" with the private or eventually privatized sectors of Canada's public health care system (Grishaber-Otto & Sinclair, 2004; Johnson, 2004a). Labour unions, in particular, have been vocal in their concern about the privatization of health facilities and the potential impact of trade agreements in the sectors where privatization has occurred, or may occur in the future.

According to the World Bank's evaluation of democratic governance, Canada is among the best-governed countries in the world. Based on numerous indicators in six broad categories, including control of corruption, effectiveness, accountability and political stability, Canada is outranked only by Sweden in the country comparison shown in Table 1.7.

Table 1.7
Worldwide governance indicator results for Canada and selected countries (percentile rank of all countries), 2010

Categories	Canada	Australia	France	Sweden	United Kingdom	United States
Voice and accountability	93.8	95.3	89.1	99.1	91.9	87.2
Political stability	81.1	74.5	70.8	88.2	58.0	56.6
Government effectiveness	96.7	96.2	89.5	98.6	92.3	90.0
Regulatory quality	96.2	95.2	87.1	96.7	97.1	90.4
Rule of law	96.2	95.3	90.5	99.5	94.8	91.5
Control of corruption	96.7	96.2	89.0	99.0	90.0	85.6
Percentile rank total	560.7	552.6	515.9	581.0	524.2	501.3
Overall percentile rank average	93.4	92.1	86.0	96.8	87.4	83.6

Source: World Bank (2011).

1.4 Health status

As Table 1.8 indicates, life expectancy has improved and mortality rates have declined since 1980. In particular, the mortality rate for adult males declined by almost 43% between 1980 and 2005, a major improvement over 25 years.

Table 1.8
Mortality and health indicators, 1980–2009 (selected years)

	1980	1990	1995	2000	2005	2009
Life expectancy at birth, total (years)	75.1	77.4	78.0	79.2	80.3	80.7
Life expectancy at birth, male (years)	71.6	74.3	75.1	76.7	78.0	78.4
Life expectancy at birth, female (years)	78.7	80.7	81.0	81.9	82.7	83.0
Total mortality rate, adult, male (per 1 000)	164.0	127.3	118.5	101.0	94.4	91.8[a]
Total mortality rate, adult, female (per 1 000)	86.3	69.7	66.9	61.1	57.1	55.4[a]

Source: World Bank (2011).
Note: [a] 2007 data.

Relative to the OECD comparators, Canada's life expectancy is at the higher end of the scale even though infant mortality and maternal mortality rates tend to be worse than those in Australia, France and (especially) Sweden. When comparing on the basis of health-adjusted life expectancy, Canada's rate is in the mid-range of the OECD comparator countries (Table 1.9).

Table 1.9

Health status, Canada and selected countries, latest available year

	Canada	Australia	France	Sweden	United Kingdom	United States
Life expectancy at birth, 2009 (years)	81	82	81	81	80	79
Infant mortality rate per 100 births, 2010	5	4	3	2	5	7
Perinatal mortality rate per 1 000 births, 2004 [a]	6	5	7	5	8	7
Maternal mortality rate per 100 000 live births, 2008	12	8	8	5	12	24
HALE (health-adjusted life expectancy) at birth, 2007	73	74	73	74	72	70

Sources: [a] WHO (2011a); WHO (2007); WHO (2010) for HALE.

As can be seen in Table 1.10, heart disease and cancer (malignant neoplasms) have alternated as the main cause of death. Among the cancers, lung cancer is the largest killer in Canada. Ischaemic heart disease (IHD) remains the most important contributor to death among the cardiovascular diseases, which includes cerebrovascular stroke, the other major killer in this category (Hu et al., 2006).

Table 1.10

Main causes of death and number of deaths per 100 000 population, 1980–2004 (selected years)

Causes of death (ICD-10 classification)	1980[a]	1990[a]	1995[a]	2000	2004
Communicable diseases	75.1	77.4	78.0	79.2	80.3
All infections and parasitic diseases (A00–B99)	6.6	9.6	11.7	20.2	24.9
Tuberculosis (A15–A19)	1.2	0.9	0.8	0.6	0.3
Sexually transmitted infections (A50–A64)	0.1	0.0	0.0	0.0	0.0
HIV/AIDS (B20–B24)	–	7.5	12.0	3.3	2.7
Noncommunicable diseases					
Circulatory diseases (100–199)	674.9	565.5	534.6	496.5	454.8
Malignant neoplasms (C00–C97)	331.0	395.1	390.9	407.4	418.8
Colon cancer (C18)	31.5	33.3	32.3	34.1	35.3
Cancer of larynx, trachea, bronchus and lung (C32–C34)	79.8	142.5	105.6	108.3	113.4
Breast cancer (C50)	28.8	34.9	32.9	31.2	30.7
Cervical cancer (C53)	3.6	3.3	2.7	2.6	2.4
Diabetes (E10–E14)	24.0	31.2	37.1	43.6	49.0
Mental and behavioural disorders (F00–F99)	5.0	21.8	34.3	38.8	42.7
Ischaemic heart diseases (I20–I25)	411.6	330.4	298.0	275.9	246.1
Cerebrovascular diseases (I60–I69)	124.7	105.3	104.8	101.0	91.3
Chronic respiratory diseases (J00–J99)	93.7	122.8	127.6	115.3	122.7
Digestive diseases (K00–K93)	58.6	52.8	51.4	52.9	54.1
External causes					
Transport accidents (V01–V99)	145.5	98.2	83.4	77.4	80.8
Suicide (X60–X84)	28.1	25.6	26.9	23.6	22.7
Signs symptoms and other ill-defined conditions (R00–R53; R55–R99)	14.2	35.3	20.2	15.7	14.7

Source: WHO (2011b).
Notes: [a] Causes of death according to ICD-9 classifications; ICD: WHO International Classification of Disease.

Overall cancer mortality for Canadian men is higher than the rates in Sweden, Australia and the United States and lower than the rates in France and the United Kingdom (Table 1.11). Female cancer mortality in Canada is the second highest among the OECD comparator countries, only slightly behind the rate in the United Kingdom. In particular, Canada's lung cancer death rates for both men and women (in tandem with the United States) are among the highest in this peer group. Although most cancer deaths are due to lung cancer, other cancers – in particular breast, prostate and colorectal cancers – are the main contributors to overall cancer morbidity (Boswell-Purdy et al. 2007).

Table 1.11
Main causes of death in Canada and selected countries by sex, latest available years

Cause of death, age-standardized rates per 100 000 people	Canada	Australia	France	Sweden	United Kingdom	United States
Year	2004	2006	2008	2008	2009	2007
Ischaemic heart disease, males	123	99	50	118	110	129
Ischaemic heart disease, females	61	52	19	58	50	68
Stroke, males	34	36	31	45	42	32
Stroke, females	29	34	22	36	39	29
All cancers, males	205	184	221	165	199	185
All cancers, females	143	115	111	125	141	130
Lung cancer, males	60	40	57	29	48	57
Lung cancer, females	36	20	14	22	30	36
Breast cancer	22.4	18.5	22.3	19.1	23.2	19.8
Prostate cancer	21.2	24.3	20.0	32.7	23.3	17.5
Road accidents, male	12.8	10.9	10.8	6.3	6.2	21.1
Road accidents, female	4.9	3.4	2.9	2.0	1.7	8.3
Suicide, males	15.7	11.9	21.6	16.1	9.8	17.1
Suicide, females	4.9	3.3	6.8	6.0	2.6	4.3

Source: OECD (2011).

While oral health has improved steadily over the last half century, there is considerable evidence that the lack of public programmes and funding has slowed potential progress in addressing dental health (Grignon et al., 2010) (Table 1.12). The Canada Health Measures Survey of 2007–2009 found that 58.8% of Canadian adolescents have one or more teeth negatively affected by dental caries (Health Canada, 2010).

Based on 2006 data (Table 1.11), both males and females in Canada had lower ischaemic heart disease (IHD) mortality rates than in Sweden, the United Kingdom and the United States. While females had a heart disease mortality rate that was equal to the rate in Australia, males had a considerably higher rate than that of Australian males. In all cases, France had the lowest IHD mortality rate. According to one study based on a national longitudinal population survey, increases in the incidence of heart disease had a strong income bias in Canada. Between 1994 and 2005, IHD incidence increased by 27% and 37% respectively in the lower income and lower middle-income categories, while it increased by 12% and 6% respectively in the upper middle and highest income categories (Lee et al., 2009).

Table 1.12

Factors influencing health status, 1990–2009 (selected years)

	1990	1995	2000	2005	2009
Alcohol consumption (litres of pure alcohol per capita, per year, 15 years and over)	8.77	7.30	7.60	7.80	8.20
Daily smokers (% of population)	28.2	24.5 [a]	22.3 [b]	17.3	17.5 [c]
Obese population (% of population aged 18 years and over with BMI>30 kg/m^2)	–	12.7	14.5	15.5	16 [d]
Measles immunizations (% of coverage among 1 year olds)	89	96	96	94	93
Diphtheria, pertussis and tetanus (DPT) immunizations (% of coverage among 1 year olds)	88	87	92	94	80

Sources: Statistics Canada (2008); OECD (2011b); WHO (2011b).
Notes: [a] 1996; [b] 2001; [c] 2008; [d] 2007; BMI: Body Mass Index.

Numerous factors influence the health of Canadians, including the consumption of alcohol and tobacco. There has been a major drop in cigarette smoking in Canada during the past two decades although the legacy of past consumption continues to be reflected in high rates of mortality attributable to smoking (Makomaski & Kaiserman, 2004). There was also a major decline in alcohol consumption in the early 1990s, although consumption has grown marginally since 1995. While national coverage for measles immunization has increased since 1990, the coverage for diphtheria, pertussis and tetanus (DPT) immunizations has seen a decline since 2005 despite earlier improvements.

Obesity rates have also increased rapidly in Canada lowering overall health status and increasing the cost of health care (Katzmarzyk & Janssen, 2004; Katzmarzyk & Mason, 2006; PHAC & CIHI, 2011). Childhood obesity has also elevated the risk of cardiovascular disease and diabetes (Ball & McCargar, 2003). While the country's obesity rate is similar to those in Australia and the United Kingdom and substantially below the rate in the United States, it is substantially above the rates in France and Sweden (Table 1.13).

Table 1.13

Percentage of the population that is overweight and obese, aged 20 years and older, Canada and selected countries, 2008

	Canada	Australia	France	Sweden	United Kingdom	United States
Obese population (% of population aged 20 years and over with BMI>30 kg/m^2)	24.3	25.1	15.6	16.6	24.9	31.8
Overweight and obese population (% of population aged 20 years and over with BMI>25 kg/m^2)	60.5	61.3	45.9	50.0	61.5	69.4

Source: WHO (2011a).

Table 1.14
Self-reported obesity by province, ages 18 years and older, 2003, 2005 and 2007–2008

	2003	2005	2007–2008
British Columbia	12.0	13.4	12.8
Alberta	15.9	16.2	19.0
Saskatchewan	20.5	21.2	23.9
Manitoba	18.8	18.5	19.6
Ontario	15.4	15.5	17.2
Quebec	14.2	14.5	15.6
New Brunswick	20.7	23.1	22.2
Nova Scotia	20.6	21.3	23.2
Prince Edward Island	21.6	23.0	23.7
Newfoundland and Labrador	20.6	24.6	25.4
Canada	15.4	15.8	17.1

Source: PHAC & CIHI (2011).

Table 1.14 illustrates the large variations in self-reported obesity among provinces. Less rural and more urbanized provinces such as British Columbia, Ontario and Quebec tend to have lower rates of obesity than more rural and sparsely populated provinces. At the same time, however, obesity is on the increase in all provinces.

Multiple indicators demonstrate that the health status of Aboriginal Canadians is well below the Canadian average. While Aboriginal health status has improved in the post-war period, relative to overall Canadian health status, a significant gap continues to persist (Frohlick, Ross & Richmond, 2006). Compared to the Canadian average, Aboriginal peoples suffer from considerably higher rates of chronic diseases, infectious diseases, injury and suicide. As with Aboriginal populations in other OECD countries such as Australia and the United States, the causes of these health disparities have long historical roots in settlement, containment and educational policies (Waldrum, Herring & Young, 2006).

2. Organization and governance

Canada has a predominantly publicly financed health system with approximately 70% of health expenditures financed through the general tax revenues of the F/P/T governments. At the same time, the governance, organization and delivery of health services is highly decentralized for at least three reasons: (1) provincial (and territorial) responsibility for the funding and delivery of most health care services; (2) the status of physicians as independent contractors; and (3) the existence of multiple organizations, from RHAs to privately governed hospitals that operate at arm's length from provincial governments (Axelsson, Marchildon & Repullo-Labrador, 2007).

The Canadian provinces and territories are responsible for administering their own tax-funded and universal hospital and medicare plans. Medically necessary hospital, diagnostic and physician services are free at the point of service for all provincial and territorial residents. Historically, the federal government played an important role in encouraging the introduction of these plans, discouraging the use of user fees and maintaining insurance portability among provinces and territories by tying contributory transfers to the upholding of these conditions. Beyond the universal basket of hospital and physician services, provincial and territorial governments subsidize or provide other health goods and services, including prescription drug coverage and long-term care and home care. In contrast to hospital and physician services, these provincial programmes generally target sub populations on the basis of age or income and can require contributory user fees.

Saskatchewan was the first province to implement a universal hospital services plan in 1947, closely followed by British Columbia and Alberta. The federal government passed the Hospital Insurance and Diagnostic Services Act in Parliament in 1957 which outlined the common conditions that provincial governments had to satisfy in order to receive shared-cost financing through federal transfers. In 1962, Saskatchewan extended coverage to include physician services and, in 1966, the federal government introduced the Medical Care Act to cost-share single-payer insurance for physician costs with provincial governments. By 1971, all provinces had universal coverage for hospital and physician services. In 1984, the federal government replaced the two previous acts with the Canada Health Act, a law that set pan-Canadian standards for hospital, diagnostic and medical care services.

Most health system planning is conducted at the provincial and territorial levels, although in some jurisdictions RHAs engage in more detailed planning of services for their defined populations. Some provincial ministries of health and RHAs are aided in their planning by provincial quality councils and specialized HTA agencies. In recent years, there has been a trend towards greater centralization in terms of reducing or eliminating RHAs. Most health professionals self-regulate under frameworks provided under provincial and territorial law.

The federal government's activities range from funding and facilitating data gathering and research to regulating prescription drugs and public health while continuing to support the national dimensions of medicare through large funding transfers to the provinces and territories. The F/P/T governments collaborate through conferences, councils and working groups comprised of ministers and deputy ministers of health. In recent years, this collaboration has been supplemented by specialized intergovernmental bodies for data collection and dissemination, HTA, patient safety, ICT and the management of blood products. Nongovernmental organizations at both federal and provincial levels influence the policy direction and management of public health care in Canada.

2.1 Overview of the health system

The federal government has jurisdiction in specific aspects of health care, including prescription drug regulation and safety; the financing and administration of a range of health benefits and services for eligible First Nations people and Inuit; and public health insurance coverage for members of the Canadian armed forces, veterans, inmates in federal penitentiaries and eligible refugee claimants. In addition, the federal government also has important responsibilities in the domains of public health, health research and health data collection (see section 2.3.2).

The provinces exercise the primary policy responsibility for funding and administering health care. In most provinces, health services are organized and delivered by geographically organized RHAs, although in some there are severe limitations on the scope of activities undertaken by RHAs (e.g. in Ontario, RHAs have no responsibility over primary health care). RHAs have been delegated by provincial ministers of health to administer hospital, institutional and community care within defined geographical areas either by delivering the services directly or by contracting with other health care organizations and providers. However, RHAs are not responsible for pharmaceutical coverage or physician remuneration. Instead, provincial ministries of health run drug plans that subsidize the cost of prescription drug therapies for residents, mainly for the poor or retired people who do not have access to PHI. Most physicians have private practices but deliver services funded and paid for by provincial ministries. Physicians receive remuneration based on fee-for-service schedules or alternative payment contracts that are periodically renegotiated with provincial ministries of health (see section 2.3.1).

Since health care is mainly a provincial responsibility, Canada's ten provinces and three territories are responsible for providing Canadians with coverage for medically necessary hospital and physician services as well as access to other health goods and services. Delivery is effected through private profit-making, private non-profit-making and public organizations as well as by physicians who receive remuneration from provincial ministries of health – 74% on a fee-for-service basis and 26% through alternative forms of remuneration. The federal government is responsible for food and drug safety, pharmaceutical patents and price regulation for branded drugs, and the enforcement of the Canada Health Act through funding transfers to the provinces. The Government of Canada also provides public health surveillance as well as funding and infrastructure for health data and health research. Through the Canada Health Transfer to the provinces and territories, the federal government has the capacity to enforce some national conditions for insured services as defined under the Canada Health Act.

Fig. 2.1 is a highly simplified overview of the governance of publicly financed health care in Canada.

Fig. 2.1
Organization of the health system in Canada

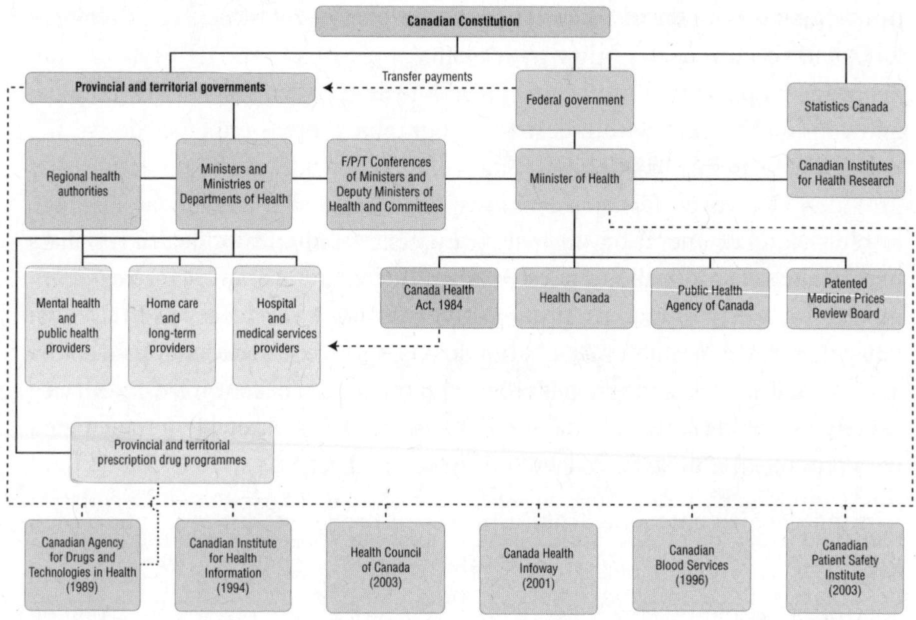

Note: Solid lines represent direct relationships of accountability while dotted lines indicate more indirect or arm's length relationships.

Canada is a constitutional federation with sovereignty, authorities and responsibilities divided between the federal government and the provincial governments. With the exception of jurisdiction over hospitals and psychiatric institutions, which the constitution assigns exclusively to the provinces, the authority over health or medical care was never explicitly addressed in the original document, which, in the 1860s, assigned powers to the central and provincial governments. As a consequence, authority can only be inferred from a number of other provisions in the constitution. Subsequent judicial decisions support the view that the provinces have primary, but not exclusive, jurisdiction over health care (Braën, 2004; Leeson, 2004). Although the three northern territories have a constitutional status that is subsidiary to the federal government, they have been delegated primary responsibility for administering public health care by the federal government.

While the funding, administration and delivery of public health care in Canada are highly decentralized (Axelsson, Marchildon & Repullo-Labrador, 2007), the federal government retains important "steering" responsibilities in terms of key dimensions of medicare through the Canada Health Act, the principles of which are upheld by provinces wanting to receive their full share of the Canada Health Transfer (see Fig. 2.1). By not taxing health benefits through employment-based insurance, the federal government also provides an implicit subsidy to encourage PHI coverage for non-medicare health services and pharmaceuticals.

2.2 Historical background

Provincial governments have a long history of providing subsidies to hospitals to admit and treat all patients irrespective of their ability to pay. The government of Ontario set the template through the Charity Aid Act of 1874 in which non-profit-making municipal, charitable and faith-based (mainly Catholic but also Protestant and Jewish) hospitals were obliged to accept some regulatory oversight – and indigent patients on the basis of medical need – in return for a per diem reimbursement. Private profit-making hospitals were excluded from this arrangement, thus restricting the growth of such hospitals in Canada. At the same time, the proliferation of municipal and non-profit-making hospitals voluntarily serving a public purpose meant that there were few state-owned and controlled hospitals (Boychuk, 1999). The major exceptions to this evolution were the provincially administered mental hospitals that emerged in the twentieth century in response to the poor state of private and nongovernmental asylums (Dyck, 2011). Cottage hospitals in the coastal fishing communities of Newfoundland as well as the inpatient institutions for the treatment of severe and chronic mental illness, tuberculosis and cancer were also run directly by some provincial governments (Grzybowski & Allen, 1999; Lawson & Noseworthy, 2009).

As was the case with hospital care of the indigent, Ontario initially led the way in facilitating financial protection in the event of illness. In 1914, the provincial government introduced worker's compensation legislation that provided medical, hospital and rehabilitation care for all entitled workers in the event of any work-related accident or injury in return for workers giving up their legal right to sue employers. This Ontario law, and the Workers' Compensation Board (WCB) that it established, became the model for the remaining provinces (Babcock, 2006). Less than two decades later, Ontario would also be the first jurisdiction to establish a province-wide medical service plan for all social assistance recipients (Naylor, 1986; Taylor, 1987).

While most provinces followed Ontario's lead in terms of targeted or categorical public health services and coverage, the provinces in western Canada laid the groundwork for the universal hospital and medical care coverage that would eventually become known as medicare. In 1916, the Government of Saskatchewan amended its municipal legislation to facilitate the establishment of hospital districts, as well as the employment of salaried doctors providing a range of health services including general medical and maternity services, and minor surgery. These hospitals and physicians served all residents of participating municipalities on the same terms and conditions (Taylor, 1987; Houston, 2002).

During the 1920s, the Government of Alberta responded to the pressure for state health insurance by establishing a commission to examine a range of policy options. The report of the Legislative Commission on Medical and Hospital Services was delivered in 1929. While this report, as well as a subsequent study, concluded that state health insurance – whether administered by the provincial government or the municipalities – was feasible, the Government of Alberta concluded that the cost to the public treasury was too high given the onset of the Great Depression of the 1930s, and delayed implementation until after World War II (Lampard, 2009).

In 1929, the Government of British Columbia appointed a Royal Commission on State Health Insurance and Medical Benefits. Delivered in 1932, the commission's report recommended a social health insurance scheme, with compulsory contributions for all employees below a threshold level of income. Although a law was passed in 1936, the scheme's implementation was postponed, and then ultimately abandoned, when the government failed to secure the cooperation of organized medicine in the province (Naylor, 1986).

As a result of the Great Depression, a growing number of Canadians were unable to pay for hospital or physician services. At the same time, government revenues fell so rapidly that it became more difficult for the provinces to consider underwriting the cost of health services. Despite this, Newfoundland introduced a state-operated cottage hospital and medical care programme to serve some of the isolated "outport" fishing communities in 1934, 15 years before it joined the Canadian federation. By the time Newfoundland (since renamed Newfoundland and Labrador) had become a province in 1949, 47% of the population was covered under the cottage hospital programme (Taylor, 1987; Lawson & Noseworthy, 2009).

The next major push for public health coverage came from the central government as part of its wartime planning and post-war reconstruction efforts (MacDougall, 2009). In the Dominion–Provincial Reconstruction Conference of 1945–1946, the federal government put forward a broad package of social security and fiscal changes, including an offer to cost-share 60% of the provincial cost of universal health insurance. The offer was ultimately rejected because of the concerns, mainly held by the Governments of Ontario and Quebec, about the administrative and tax arrangements that would accompany the comprehensive social security programme. The failure of this conference forced a more piecemeal approach to the introduction of universal health coverage in the post-war years.

In 1947, the Saskatchewan Government implemented a universal hospital services plan popularly known as "hospitalization". Unlike private insurance policies, no limitation was placed on the number of "entitlement days" as long as the hospital services rendered were medically necessary and no distinction was made between basic services and optional extras. In addition to hospital services, coverage included X-rays, laboratory services and some prescription drugs used on an inpatient basis. These design features did much to eliminate the possibility of a parallel tier of private hospital insurance. Saskatchewan was financially aided by the federal government with the introduction of national health grants in 1948 (Johnson, 2004b). In addition to providing money for new hospital construction, these grants helped to fund provincial initiatives in public health, mental health, venereal disease, tuberculosis and general health surveys (Taylor, 1987).

In 1949, the Government of British Columbia implemented a universal hospital insurance scheme based on the Saskatchewan model. One year later, the Government of Alberta introduced its own hospitalization scheme through subsidies paid to those municipalities that agreed to provide public hospital coverage to residents. Both programmes encountered challenges. In British Columbia, the difficulty of premium collection led to a revamping of the programme after a new administration was elected in 1952 (Marchildon & O'Byrne, 2009). In Alberta, the partial and voluntary nature of the initiative meant that on the eve of the introduction of national hospitalization in 1957, 25% of the population still did not have hospital insurance (Marchildon, 2009).

In 1955, the Government of Ontario announced its willingness to implement public coverage for hospital and diagnostic services if the federal government would share the cost with the province. One year later, the federal government agreed in principle to the proposal, and passed the Hospital Insurance and

Diagnostic Services Act in parliament in 1957. This law set out the common conditions that provincial governments would have to satisfy in order to receive shared-cost financing through federal transfers. One year later in 1958, the provinces of Saskatchewan, British Columbia, Alberta, Manitoba and Newfoundland agreed to work within the federal framework. By 1959, Ontario, Nova Scotia, New Brunswick and Prince Edward Island also joined. Quebec did not agree until 1961, shortly after the election of a government dedicated to modernizing the provincial welfare state (Taylor, 1987) (Table 2.1).

With the introduction of federal cost-sharing for universal hospitalization, the Saskatchewan Government was financially able to proceed with universal coverage for physician services. However, the introduction of the prepaid, publicly administered medical care insurance plan triggered a bitter, province-wide, doctors' strike in 1962 that lasted for 23 days. The strike officially ended with a compromise known as the Saskatoon Agreement in which the nature and mechanism of payment emphasized the contractual autonomy of physicians from the provincial government, and fee-for-service as the dominant method of payment (Badgley & Wolfe, 1967; Marchildon & Schrijvers, 2011).

In 1964, the Royal Commission on Health Services, commonly known as the Hall Commission, delivered its report to the Prime Minister. This federal commission had been established in the wake of the polarized debate in Saskatchewan about the merits of single-payer, universal medical care insurance compared with the state providing targeted subsidies for the purchase of private insurance as championed by Alberta and organized medicine. Ultimately, the Hall Commission leaned in favour of the Saskatchewan model, and recommended that the federal government encourage other provinces to implement universal medical care insurance through conditional grants (Canada, 1964). In 1966, the federal government passed the Medical Care Act with federal cost-sharing transfers to begin flowing in 1968 to those provinces that conformed to the four conditions of universality, public administration, comprehensiveness and portability. By 1972, all the provinces and territories had implemented universal coverage for medical care to complement their existing universal coverage for hospital care. This federal–provincial system of narrow but deep coverage would become known as medicare (Marchildon, 2009).

The 1970s marked a period of rapid expansion of public coverage and subsidies for health services well beyond hospital and medical care by the provinces and territories. These included prescription drug plans as well as subsidies for long-term care. However, lacking any national principles or federal funding, these initiatives varied considerably across the country, depending on the fiscal capacity and policy ambitions of individual provinces and territories.

Table 2.1
Chronology of the evolution of public health care in Canada, 1946–1984

1946	Federal health insurance proposals rejected by majority of provinces in Dominion-Provincial Reconstruction Conference
1947	Saskatchewan implements universal hospital insurance
1948	Federal health minister introduces Hospital Grants Program and British Columbia implements universal hospital insurance (British Columbia Hospital Insurance Services)
1950	Alberta introduces a provincially subsidized but municipally administered and financed hospital insurance
1955	Canadian Medical Association passes resolution officially opposing universal health care
1957	Federal government enacts the Hospital Insurance and Diagnostic Services Act that cost-shares hospital insurance with provinces
1961	Federal government establishes the Royal Commission on Health Services (Hall Commission) to examine feasibility of national medical care insurance
1962	Saskatchewan implements universal medical care insurance after a province-wide, 23-day doctors' strike
1963	Alberta Government introduces alternative to Saskatchewan's universal plan based on subsidizing purchase of private insurance plans
1964	Hall Commission report recommends universal medical care insurance based on Saskatchewan model
1965	British Columbia introduces multi-payer medical care insurance involving non-profit-making insurance carriers
1966	Federal government introduces Medical Care Act to cost-share single-payer universal medical care insurance with provincial governments
1968	Implementation of universal medical care insurance on national basis through federal cost-sharing: Saskatchewan and British Columbia qualify; followed by Alberta, Manitoba, Ontario, Nova Scotia and Newfoundland in 1969, Quebec and Prince Edward Island in 1970; and New Brunswick in 1971
1974	Government of Canada publishes Lalonde Report on factors beyond medical care such as lifestyle, environment and biology that determine health outcomes
1977	Established Programs Financing (EPF) with block transfer replaces federal cost-sharing with provinces for medicare
1980	Hall's medicare check-up report on medicare to federal government concerning impact of user fees and extra billing
1984	Federal government, led by Health Minister Monique Bégin, introduces the Canada Health Act which discourages extra billing and user fees for physician and hospital services

During the same period, the federal government initiated much new thinking concerning the basic determinants of health beyond medical care, including biological factors and lifestyle choices, as well as environmental, social and economic conditions. In 1974, the Canadian Minister of Health, Marc Lalonde, summarized this new approach in a report – *A New Perspective on the Health of Canadians* (Health and Welfare Canada, 1974). Emphasizing the upstream determinants of health, the Lalonde Report influenced subsequent studies and provided some of the intellectual foundation for the "wellness" reforms introduced by provincial governments in the early 1990s (Boychuk, 2009).

In 1984, the federal government replaced the Hospital Insurance and Diagnostic Services Act and the Medical Care Act with the Canada Health Act, a law that required the federal government to deduct (dollar-for-dollar) from a provincial government's share of Established Programs Financing (EPF) the value of all extra billing and user fees permitted in that province (Taylor, 1987). The origins of the Canada Health Act can be traced to the federal government's concern that, despite the stipulation in the Medical Care Act that provincial plans must allow user fees to "impede or preclude" any "reasonable access to insured services", some provincial governments had increasingly permitted the imposition of patient user fees by hospitals and physicians by the late 1970s (see section 3.3.3). In addition to incorporating the four original funding criteria – public administration, comprehensiveness, universality and portability – from its earlier laws, the federal government added a fifth criterion – accessibility – to reinforce the view that access should not be impeded by user fees. At the same time, the federal government made it clear that provincial governments that eliminated all user fees within three years of the introduction of the new law would have their deductions reimbursed at the end of that period. By 1988, extra billing and user fees had been virtually eliminated for all insured services under the Canada Health Act (Bégin, 1988).

Table 2.2

Five funding criteria of the Canada Health Act (1984)

Criteria	Each provincial health care insurance plan must:
Public Administration Section 8	Be administered and operated on a non-profit-making basis by a public authority
Comprehensiveness Section 9	Cover all insured health services provided by hospitals, physicians or dentists (surgical dental services that require a hospital setting) and, where the law of a province permits, similar or additional services rendered by other health care practitioners
Universality Section 10	Ensure entitlement to all insured health services on uniform terms and conditions
Portability Section 11	Not impose a minimum period of residence, or waiting period, in excess of three months for new residents; pay for insured health services for its own residents if temporarily visiting another province (or country in the case of non-elective services) with reimbursement paid at the home rate of province or territory; and cover the waiting period for those residents moving to another province after which the new province of residence assumes responsibility for health care coverage (see section 2.9.6 for application outside of Canada)
Accessibility Section 12	Not impede or preclude, either directly or indirectly, whether by charges made to insured persons or otherwise, reasonable access to insured health services

Source: Health Canada (2011).

While the five criteria of the Canada Health Act (summarized in Table 2.2) started out as funding conditions, over time they have come to represent the principles and values that underpin Canadian medicare. After extensive national consultations in 2001 and 2002, the Commission on the Future of

Health Care in Canada concluded that the five principles had "stood the test of time" and continued "to reflect the values of Canadians" (Romanow, 2002, p.60). At the same time, the Romanow Commission recommended increasing the modest conditionality of the Canada Health Act and adding a sixth principle of accountability. However, most provincial governments oppose additional conditionality of federal transfers, if only because it would reduce their own fiscal flexibility and control over budgetary priority setting, and the federal government has made no changes to the Canada Health Act since its introduction.

In addition to providing financial security, universal medicare appears to have had positive outcomes in reducing health disparities since it was first introduced. In a study covering 25 years following the introduction of universal medical care insurance in Canada, James et al. (2007) demonstrated a major reduction in disparity as measured by the rates of death amenable to medical care.

2.3 Organization

2.3.1 The provincial and territorial level

Each province and territory has legislation governing the administration of a single-payer system for universal hospital and physician services that has come to be known as medicare (Marchildon, 2009). In addition to paying for hospital care, either directly or through funding for RHAs, provinces also set rates of remuneration for physicians that are negotiated with provincial medical associations (RHAs' budgets do not include physician services). Provincial governments also administer a variety of long-term care subsidies and services as well as prescription drug plans that provide varying degrees of coverage to residents. These non-medicare services have grown over time relative to hospital and physician services and constituted roughly 40% of total provincial and territorial health expenditures in 2011, compared with 23% in 1975 (CIHI, 2011e).

Provincial and territorial ministers of health are responsible for the laws and regulations for the administration of universal coverage for medically necessary hospital and physician services. In some jurisdictions, there are two separate laws, one pertaining to inpatient services and the other to medical services, while in other jurisdictions, both have been combined in a single law (see section 9.3). In provinces and territories with RHAs, some of the minister of health's authority and responsibility for the health system is delegated to RHAs, which are responsible for allocating resources for a range of health services for populations within a geographically defined region.

Regionalization combines devolution of funding from provincial ministries of health to the RHAs with a centralization of governance and administration from individual health care facilities and organizations to RHAs. In most provinces, RHAs act both as providers and purchasers of hospital care and long-term care as well as other services delegated by provincial law. In Ontario, RHAs known as LHINs (Local Health Integration Networks) do not provide services directly; instead, they allocate resources among hospitals and other independent health organizations. While in some cases RHAs facilitated horizontal integration, in particular the consolidation of hospitals, the main purpose of regionalization was to gain the benefits of vertical integration. By coordinating or integrating facilities and providers across a number of health sectors, RHAs were expected to improve the continuity of care and reduce costs by encouraging more upstream preventive care and, where appropriate, substituting potentially lower-cost home, community and institutional services for more expensive hospital care. With funding from provincial ministries of health, RHAs are expected to allocate health resources in a manner that optimally serves the needs of their respective populations. However, no provincial government has delegated physician remuneration, including remuneration for family doctors who are responsible for the majority of primary care provision, or the administration of public prescription drug plans to RHAs (Lewis & Kouri, 2004) (Table 2.3).

2.3.2 The federal level

This section and the following two (2.3.3 and 2.3.4) provide a catalogue of federal, intergovernmental and nongovernmental national agencies and associations relevant to the health care system and their duties (see also Fig. 2.1).

Table 2.3
Regionalization in the provinces and territories

	RHAs first established (year)	Number of RHAs when first established	Number of RHAs in 2011
British Columbia	1997	52	5
Alberta	1994	17	1
Saskatchewan	1992	32	13
Manitoba	1997	12	11
Ontario	2005	14	14
Quebec	1989	18	18
New Brunswick	1992	8	2
Nova Scotia	1996	4	9
Prince Edward Island	1993	6	1
Newfoundland and Labrador	1994	6	6
Northwest Territories	1997	8	8

Sources: Axelsson, Marchildon & Repullo-Labrador (2007) and current provincial and territorial ministry websites consulted in November 2011 (see section 9.2).
Notes: Year of RHA establishment based on calendar year in which law establishing regionalization was passed; jurisdictions with one RHA have separated RHA governance and mandate from ministry of health governance and mandate, similar to other regionalized jurisdictions.

While the provinces have the primary governance responsibility for most public health care services, the federal government plays a key role in setting pan-Canadian standards for hospital, diagnostic and medical care services through the Canada Health Act and the Canada Health Transfer (see section 3.3.3). The federal department of health – Health Canada – is responsible for ensuring that the provincial and territorial governments are adhering to the five criteria of the Canada Health Act. Although conditional transfers are a common policy tool in most federations, the use of the federal spending power in health care has been more controversial in Canada, in large part because of the desire of some provincial governments and policy advocates for an even greater degree of fiscal and administrative decentralization (Marchildon, 2004; Boessenkool, 2010).

While provincial and territorial governments must provide universally insured services to all registered Indians and recognized Inuit residents, the First Nations and Inuit Health Branch of Health Canada provides these citizens supplemental coverage for "non-insured health benefits" (NIHB) such as prescription drugs, dental care and vision care as well as medical transportation to access medicare services not provided on-reserve or in the community of residence. In addition, Health Canada and the PHAC provide a number of population health and community health programmes in First Nation and Inuit communities. Health Canada is also responsible for regulating the safety and efficacy of therapeutic products, including medical devices, pharmaceuticals and natural health products, and for ensuring food and consumer product safety. Data and patent protection for drug products are also administered by Health Canada under the Food and Drugs Act and the Patented Medicines (Notice of Compliance) Regulations under the Patent Act.

Established as a department in 2004, the PHAC performs a broad array of public health functions including infectious disease control, surveillance, emergency preparedness leading national immunization and vaccination initiatives, as well as coordinating or administrating programmes for health promotion, illness prevention and travel health. As part of its mandate, PHAC is responsible for regionally distributed centres and laboratories including the biosafety facilities at the National Microbiology Laboratory.

An arm's length quasi-judicial body – the Patented Medicine Prices Review Board (PMPRB) – regulates the factory-gate price (defined as the price at which pharmaceutical manufacturers sell to hospitals, pharmacies and other wholesalers) of patented drugs. Established in 1987, the PMPRB was mandated to act as a watchdog on patented drug prices at the same time that the federal government enhanced monopoly protection for new pharmaceuticals under the Patent Act. It is important to note that the PMPRB does not have jurisdiction over the prices charged by wholesalers or pharmacies, or over the professional fees of pharmacists. Although the PMPRB has no mandate to regulate generic drug prices, it does report annually to parliament on the price trends of all drugs (see section 2.8.4).

In addition, the federal government plays a critical role in health research through the funding of the Canadian Institutes of Health Research (CIHR). In 2000, the CIHR replaced the Medical Research Council as the country's national health research funding agency. The CIHR is made up of 13 "virtual" institutes that provide research funding for Aboriginal peoples' health; ageing; cancer; circulatory and respiratory health; gender and health; genetics; health services and policy; human development, child and youth health; infection and immunity; musculoskeletal health and arthritis; neurosciences, mental health and addiction; nutrition, metabolism and diabetes; and population and public health. While the majority of CIHR-sponsored research is investigator driven, approximately 30% of CIHR-funded research is based on strategic objectives set by the organization's governing council. The federal minister of health is responsible to parliament for CIHR and the government's stated objective of making Canada one of the five leading health research nations in the world.

This research activity is supported by an extensive infrastructure for health data provided by Statistics Canada through five-year censuses as well as a number of health surveys. Long recognized as one of the world's premier statistical agencies, Statistics Canada was a pioneer in the gathering of health statistics as well as in the development of indicators of health status and the determinants of health. Data collection has been extended considerably through Statistics Canada's partnership with the Canadian Institute for Health Information (CIHI) (see section 2.3.3).

The federal government also provides the majority of funding for major research initiatives that are governed independently, including Genome Canada and the Canadian Health Services Research Foundation (CHSRF)[1]. Genome Canada's objective is to make Canada a world leader in research capable of isolating disease predisposition and developing better diagnostic tools and prevention strategies. CHSRF focuses on research in health services aimed at improving health care organization, administration and delivery as well as acting as knowledge brokers between the research and decision-making communities.

2.3.3 The intergovernmental level

As a decentralized state operating in an environment of increasing health policy interdependence, the F/P/T governments rely heavily on both direct and arm's length intergovernmental instruments to facilitate and coordinate policy and programme areas (Marchildon, 2010). The direct instruments are F/P/T advisory councils and committees which report to the Conference of F/P/T Deputy Ministers of Health, which, in turn, report to the Conference of F/P/T Ministers of Health (O'Reilly, 2001). The more arm's length intergovernmental instruments, most of which have been established very recently, are intergovernmental non-profit-making corporations funded and partially governed by the sponsoring governments.

The Conference of F/P/T Ministers of Health is co-chaired by the federal minister and a provincial minister of health selected on a rotating basis. This committee is mirrored by the Conference of F/P/T Deputy Ministers of Health with an identical chair arrangement. In order to conduct their work in priority areas of concern, the ministers and deputy ministers of health have established, reorganized and disbanded various advisory committees and task forces over time, including those on health delivery and human resources, information and emerging technologies, population health and health security as well as

[1] At the time of press CHSRF was renamed the Canadian Foundation for Healthcare Improvement.

governance and accountability. They have also established more arm's length and special purpose intergovernmental bodies (illustrated at the bottom of Fig. 2.1) to support work in priority areas determined by F/P/T governments. In most cases, the federal government provides a significant share of the funding.

The Canadian Agency for Drugs and Technologies in Health (CADTH) was first established under the name of the Canadian Coordinating Office for Health Technology Assessment. Its mandate is to encourage the appropriate use of health technology by influencing decision-makers through the collection, creation and dissemination of HTA of new medical technologies and pharmaceutical therapies. Given the existence of provincial HTA organizations, this also means that CADTH coordinates the dissemination of existing studies throughout the country as well as original HTAs in areas not covered by the provincial agencies. CADTH is funded by Health Canada and by the provinces and territories (in proportion to population) with the exception of Quebec. In 2003, CADTH launched the Common Drug Review (CDR), a single, pan-Canadian process for reviewing new drugs and making formulary recommendations to the government members of CADTH (Menon & Stafinski, 2009).

Established in 1994, the Canadian Institute for Health Information (CIHI) was a response to the desire of F/P/T governments for a nationally coordinated approach to gathering and analysing their respective financial and administrative data. Its core functions include identifying and defining national health indicators and frameworks, coordinating the development and maintenance of pan-Canadian data standards, developing and managing F/P/T health databases and registries, and disseminating health data through research reports. By 2011, CIHI was maintaining a total of 27 databases and clinical registries, including the National Health Expenditure Database, the National Physician Database, the Hospital Morbidity Database, the Discharge Abstract Database and the National Prescription Drug Utilization and Information Systems Database. Approximately 80% of CIHI's funding comes from Health Canada and the remaining funds from provincial governments. CIHI also has an ongoing partnership with Statistics Canada, as well as a strong advisory relationship with the Conference of F/P/T Deputy Ministers of Health through its 16-member board of directors.

Canada Health Infoway is a product of the 2000 First Ministers' Accord on Health Care Renewal and the priority assigned by F/P/T ministries of health to the development of electronic health records (EHRs) using compatible standards. Since its creation in 2001, Infoway has been allocated C$2.1 billion in federal government funding to work with provincial and territorial governments to support the development and implementation of electronic health technologies – including electronic health and medical records – and electronic public health surveillance systems. Similar to CIHI, all F/P/T governments including Quebec are members of Canada Health Infoway. The 2003 First Ministers' Accord on Health Care Renewal provided additional funding for Canada Health Infoway to stimulate new telehealth initiatives. Infoway acts as a national umbrella organization to facilitate the interoperability of existing F/P/T electronic health information initiatives. Infoway released a common framework and standards blueprint, first in 2003 and subsequently revised in 2006, for EHR development (Canada Health Infoway, 2003, 2006).

The origins of the Health Council of Canada can be found in the final recommendations of the Romanow Commission and the Senate Committee reports of 2002, although the general idea of establishing a pan-Canadian, arm's length policy advisory body has a longer history (Adams, 2001; Romanow, 2002; Senate of Canada, 2002). The Health Council was established in 2003 without the participation of the provincial governments of Quebec and Alberta, although Alberta subsequently joined in 2012. The board of the Health Council is chaired by an individual nominated by consensus of the participating F/P/T ministers of health. The remaining members of the board are based on the nominations of each participating government. The mandate of the Health Council of Canada is to monitor and report on the implementation of commitments made in F/P/T health accords.

The Canadian Patient Safety Institute (CPSI) was created a year after its establishment was recommended by the nongovernmental National Steering Committee on Patient Safety (2002), an idea that was endorsed one year later by first ministers (CICS, 2003). Funded largely by the federal government and governed by a board made up of individuals appointed by participating governments, CPSI was mandated to provide a leadership role in building a culture of patient safety and quality improvement in Canada through promotion of best practices and advising on effective strategies to improve patient safety.

Canadian Bloods Services (CBS) is a non-profit-making charitable organization established by the provinces and territories in the late 1990s in response to a tainted blood controversy and the exit of the Canadian Red Cross from the management of blood products and services in Canada (Rock, 2000). Although funded by the participating provinces and territories, CBS is governed at arm's length from all participating provincial–territorial (P/T) governments.

While CBS's board members are nominated by P/T ministers of health, civil servants are not permitted on the board. Quebec is not a participating member of CBS and instead has it own blood products and services agency – Héma-Québec.

F/P/T governments collaborate extensively with civil society partners in a number of other pan-Canadian health initiatives, including the Canadian Partnership Against Cancer Corporation and the Pan-Canadian Public Health Network. Through the Council of the Federation, provincial and territorial governments recently created a Health Care Innovation Working Group made up of all P/T ministers of health. In 2012, this Working Group was mandated to examine human resources management, provider scope of practice and clinical practice guidelines in order to identify and learn from innovative initiatives in Canada.

2.3.4 Nongovernmental national agencies and associations

Canadian health care programmes and policies are highly influenced by a number of nongovernmental organizations including health services associations, professional organizations such as regulatory bodies, protective associations, trade unions, industry associations, and patient and disease advocacy associations. Many are organized as provincial associations – one study found that there were 244 such organizations operating in Ontario alone (Wiktorowicz et al., 2003). A number of these provincial bodies have national umbrella organizations that play an important role in facilitating and coordinating the memberships' pan-Canadian initiatives. Some of the larger or more influential of these national organizations are described below.

Accreditation Canada is a voluntary, nongovernmental organization that accredits hospitals, health facilities and RHAs. Funded by the organizations it accredits, Accreditation Canada also conducts reviews and assessments of health facilities and regional health systems with recommendations for improvements. First established in 1958, Accreditation Canada has expanded its mandate beyond acute care hospitals to psychiatric facilities (1964), long-term care institutions (1978), rehabilitation facilities (1985), community-based health services (1995) and home care services (1996).[2] There has been some debate in Canada as to whether accreditation should be made compulsory, and two provinces – Quebec and Alberta – have moved to mandatory accreditation with a third – Manitoba – considering a similar change (Nicklin,

[2] Accreditation Canada's name changes reflect its expanding mandate: in 1958, it was first incorporated as the Canadian Council on Hospital Accreditation; 30 years later (1988), the name was changed to the Canadian Council on Health Facilities Accreditation; in 1995, it was reincorporated as the Canadian Council on Health Services Accreditation; and finally, in 2008, it became Accreditation Canada.

2011). Connected to this debate is the question of whether voluntary (or even compulsory) accreditation actually serves to improve health system quality and safety or whether it is a "sterile administrative ritual" (Lozeau, 1999). In a study comparing France, which has had a compulsory accreditation regime since 1996, and Canada, with its predominantly voluntary approach, Touati & Pomey (2009) found that both systems have contributed to quality and safety improvements although in very different ways.

Health provider organizations, in particular physician organizations and, more recently, nurse organizations, have played a major role in shaping health care policy in Canada (see section 9.2.5). Other provider organizations including those representing dentists, optometrists, pharmacists, psychologists, medical technologists and many others are also more active in attempting to influence future health system reforms.

The Canadian Medical Association (CMA) is the umbrella national organization for physicians, including consultants – known as specialists in Canada – and general practitioners. In addition to lobbying for its members' interests, the CMA also conducts an active policy research agenda and publishes the biweekly *CMAJ (Canadian Medication Association Journal)* as well as six more specialized medical journals. The 12 P/T medical associations (Nunavut is not represented) are self-governing divisions within the CMA. These P/T bodies are responsible for negotiating physician remuneration and working conditions with P/T ministries of health, except in Quebec where negotiations are carried out by two bodies representing specialists and general practitioners. While the CMA is not involved directly in such bargaining, it does – when called upon – provide advice and expertise to the P/T associations.

The role of the CMA and, in particular, its provincial divisions, must be separated from the regulatory role of the provincial colleges of physicians and surgeons. The latter are responsible for the licensing of physicians, the development and enforcement of standards of practice, investigation of patient complaints against members for alleged breaches of ethical or professional conduct and standards of practice as well as enforcement. As is the case with most professions in Canada, physicians are responsible for regulating themselves within the framework of provincial laws. A national body, the Royal College of Physicians and Surgeons of Canada (RCPSC), restricts its function to overseeing and regulating postgraduate medical education.

The Canadian Nurses Association (CNA) is a federation of 11 P/T registered nurses (RN) organizations with approximately 144 000 members as of 2011.[3] Some of the provincial organizations such as the Registered Nurses Association of Ontario (RNAO) carry considerable political influence within their respective jurisdictions. The CNA and its provincial affiliates have also played a major role in carving out a larger role for nurse practitioners in Canada. P/T nurses associations are not involved in collective bargaining with the provinces. This is the function of the various unions in the provinces and territories representing RNs and licensed practical nurses (LPNs). The Canadian Federation of Nurses Unions (CFNU) is an umbrella organization for all provincial and territorial nurses' unions with the exception of Quebec.

There are numerous civil society groups at the pan-Canadian level with the chief objective being to mobilize support and funding for both general and specific health care causes (see section 9.26). Some examples of organizations with a more general policy advocacy role, sometimes combined with a research mandate, include the Canadian Healthcare Association (formerly the Canadian Hospital Association), the Canadian Health Coalition, the Canadian Public Health Association (CPHA), the Canadian Women's Health Network, the Canadian Home Care Association and the Canadian Hospice Palliative Care Association among many others. Other charitable organizations promote a greater public focus on particular diseases or health conditions through advocacy, information and advice for affected individuals and their caregivers. Many of these organizations have charitable status and provide funding for research in their respective areas. Some of the larger of these pan-Canadian charities are identified in section 9.2.6.

Finally, there are industry associations that represent profit-making interests in health care. These include organizations such as the Canadian Generic Pharmaceuticals Association, Canada's Research-Based Pharmaceutical Companies, and the Canadian Life and Health Insurance Association.

2.4 Decentralization and centralization

While Canada is a highly decentralized federation with a mixed model of public and private health delivery, the administration of health care has become more centralized as a result of large-scale administrative reforms enacted by P/T governments during the past two decades. When regionalization first occurred,

[3] The association of nurses of Quebec (Ordre des infirmières et infirmiers du Québec – OIIQ) is not a member of the CNA, while there is a single association for nurses in Nunavut and the Northwest Territories.

it involved both decentralization and centralization. While P/T ministries of health delegated considerable administrative decision-making to quasi-public RHAs, in many (but not all) cases this structural change also involved the abolishment of a number of more local (municipal and quasi-public) health care organizations and their boards of directors, with these organizations folded into the RHAs (see section 2.3.1).

Since 2001, there has been a trend towards increased centralization in terms of reducing the number of RHAs, thereby increasing the geographical and population size of individual RHAs. In 2005, the same year that Ontario introduced its particular brand of regionalization, the government of Prince Edward Island eliminated its two RHAs (Axelsson, Marchildon & Repullo-Labrador, 2007). In 2008, Alberta disbanded its nine RHAs in favour of a single RHA in an ambitious effort to gain economies of scale and scope by creating what was in effect a single health management organization for its more than 3.5 million residents. As a single RHA, Alberta Health Services has some operational autonomy from the provincial ministry of health (Duckett, 2010; Donaldson, 2010).

At the same time, however, the delivery of the majority of primary health services is private and therefore decentralized. The vast majority of family physicians are profit-making professional contractors and are not directly employed by either the RHAs or P/T ministries of health. While hospitals are divided in ownership – some are owned by RHAs while others remain private, largely non-profit-making, corporations – specialist physicians who provide acute services are also private, independent contractors. In most provinces, a significant number of consultants (specialist physicians) have been incorporated as professional corporations mainly to increase their after-tax income. Most services supporting primary and acute care, including ambulance, blood and laboratory services as well as the ancillary hospital services (e.g. laundry and food), are private. Long-term care facilities are divided between public (P/T and local government) and private (profit-making and non-profit-making). The majority of dental care, vision care, psychology and rehabilitation services are privately funded and delivered by independent professionals.

2.5 Planning

As a consequence of the constitutional division of powers in Canada and the relatively decentralized nature of health administration and delivery, there is no single agency responsible for system-wide national planning.

Instead, pan-Canadian initiatives are often the product of intergovernmental agreements, committees and agencies that do a limited amount of high-level strategic planning, most often on a sector-by-sector basis such as HTA, EHRs, and administrative data collection and dissemination. There are two notable exceptions to this: the first is the F/P/T Councils of Ministers of Health and Deputy Ministers of Health and their respective working groups; and the second is the Health Council of Canada, although its mandate is limited to producing progress reports on the health reform priorities identified by participating governments (see section 2.3.3).

Most system-wide planning is actually done within the provincial and territorial ministries of health and each provincial and territorial ministry has a policy and planning unit. In regionalized provinces and territories, some planning has been delegated to RHAs but P/T ministries continue to be responsible for major new capital (e.g. hospital) as well as some infrastructure planning. Health human resource (HHR) planning tends to be divided between the ministries and RHAs, with the responsibilities varying among provinces. In smaller non-regionalized jurisdictions such as Prince Edward Island, Yukon and Nunavut, HHR planning is done at the ministry level. Due to the mobility of health professionals in Canada, P/T ministries and RHAs are sensitive to changes in remuneration, working conditions and regulatory requirements in other jurisdictions. In the 2000s, a number of provinces established health research agencies and health quality councils with a mandate to help improve health system processes and outcomes as well as to influence, if not reshape, physician practice and clinical decision-making.

Perhaps the single most important initiative in system-wide planning has been the creation of RHAs by provincial governments. Operating at an intermediate level between health ministries and individual providers, RHAs have a legal mandate to plan the coordination and continuity of care among a host of health care organizations and providers within a defined geographical area (Denis, 2004; Marchildon, 2006). While a broad strategic direction is set by P/T health ministries, detailed planning and coordination is actually done at the RHA level. RHAs set their priorities through annual budgets (occasionally supplemented by multi-year plans) that are submitted to provincial health ministries. Some budget submissions are required before the ministry budget is finalized while others are submitted only after funding is announced in the provincial budget, with each approach having different implications for the planning process (McKillop, 2004).

There has been a marked improvement in risk management and disaster planning since an earlier, and largely negative, assessment of the readiness of Canadian hospitals and health care professionals working in hospitals to deal with a national emergency (Government of Canada, 2002). According to the federal government's current emergency response plan, Health Canada and the PHAC share responsibility for coordinating the public health and health care emergency response dimensions of any national emergency or an international emergency with a domestic impact (Government of Canada, 2011). In the event of a nuclear or radiological emergency, Health Canada is responsible for coordinating any response with affected P/T health ministries and other affected parties (Health Canada, 2002), while the Canadian Food Inspection Agency is responsible for coordinating the response to any major outbreak of a food-related illness (e.g. bovine spongiform encephalopathy). The CBS and, in Quebec, Héma Québec, are responsible for ensuring adequate inventories of fresh blood and frozen plasma to prepare for an emergency.

Health Canada and the Canadian International Development Agency are responsible for most of the health-related international development assistance. The majority of this flows to lower income countries in Latin America and the Caribbean islands as a result of Canada's membership in the Pan American Health Organization. In the fiscal year 2009–2010, Health Canada alone distributed C$13.4 million in health-related development assistance.

2.6 Intersectorality

Some provincial governments have experimented with intersectoral cabinet committees or committees of senior officials to address cross-cutting health issues and policies, in particular emphasizing the determinants of health and illness prevention. For example, the Government of Manitoba established a Healthy Child Committee of Cabinet – one of four permanent cabinet committees – to encourage intersectoral health initiatives to address the health of children from the prenatal period through the preschool years.

In British Columbia, the government set up an intersectoral committee of senior officials (assistant deputy ministers) to pursue health promotion and chronic disease prevention throughout the province. In addition, ActNow BC is a major health promotion partnership between the provincial government, the voluntary sector and civil society that targets six population health areas: physical activity; diet, schools; work environments; communities; pregnancy; and tobacco use (HCC, 2010b).

In Quebec, the Public Health Act of 2001 empowers the Minister of Health and Social Services to initiate intersectoral actions that reflect policies favourable to the health of the provincial population. The Act also requires that the legislative and regulatory proposals from all other departments and agencies in the Quebec Government be subjected to a mandatory health impact assessment. In Ontario, the provincial government is exploring a "health in all policy" approach that appears to have originated in Finland (Ståhl et al., 2006). This approach, if implemented, would embed a health equity assessment tool in the development of all policies in the Ontario Government (HCC, 2010b).

While there have been a number of intersectoral health initiatives in Canada, few have set targets with clearly defined objectives within specified time frames. In addition, these initiatives have not generally been accompanied by a systematic evaluation of processes and outcomes. While these are features that the Canadian initiatives share with similar intersectoral initiatives in other countries (PHAC, 2008), there is an opportunity for more specific target setting and systematic evaluation in future intersectoral initiatives.

2.7 Health information management

To support system-wide planning, provincial governments have invested in health ICT infrastructures with plans to create EHRs for all provincial residents. As befits its federal character, Canada has a plurality of information systems in place for the collection, reporting and analysis of health data.

2.7.1 Data and information systems

At the P/T level, governments have been collecting detailed administrative data since the introduction of universal hospital and medical insurance plans. At the federal level, Statistics Canada has been collecting population health data through both the national census taken every five years and large-sample health surveys, including the Canadian Community Health Survey (CCHS), a cross-sectional patient self-report survey, and the Canadian Health Measures Survey (CHMS), a direct measure survey of the Canadian population. Statistics Canada is governed by a legislative framework – the Statistics Act – that makes the provision of basic census data compulsory while protecting individual privacy and confidentiality. However, the Government of Canada decided, as of the 2011 Census, to eliminate the compulsory long-form census that had asked 20% of respondents additional health questions in favour of a voluntary survey.

At the intergovernmental level, CIHI coordinates the collection and dissemination of health data, much of which is administrative data provided by the provinces and territories. CIHI works with F/P/T governments in establishing and maintaining data definitions and quality standards. The agency also works with provider organizations in maintaining databases, including physician and hospital discharge databases. In a unique provincial arrangement, the Manitoba Centre for Health Policy (MCHP) at the University of Manitoba maintains the administrative database for the ministry of health. Based on a long-standing contract with the provincial ministry, the MCHP analyses the data and publishes analytical reports and peer-reviewed journal articles based on the administrative data.

Since the 1990s, privacy has emerged as a major issue in health data collection and dissemination. The collection and use of personal health information are inherently privacy-intrusive activities in which judgements are continually made as to whether the public good of obtaining, analysing and using such data outweighs the potential intrusion on an individual's confidentiality and privacy. Since jurisdiction over health information is shared among F/P/T governments, the result is a patchwork of health information and privacy laws in Canada. These laws sometimes address three issues – privacy, confidentiality and security – in the same legislation, or at other times in separate laws within the same jurisdiction.

At the federal level, four major laws govern privacy. The Personal Information Protection and Electronic Documents Act (PIPEDA) applies to personal health data that are collected, used or disclosed in the course of commercial activities that cross provincial and territorial borders. The Privacy Act requires informed consent before information is collected or used. Within the limits of strict legal protection for individual confidentiality, the Statistics Act permits Statistics Canada to collect and disseminate health and other data. At the same time, the Access to Information Act requires that public information held by the federal government or its agencies be made publicly available unless it is specifically exempt.

At the P/T level, most jurisdictions have general laws in place to protect privacy and confidentiality, although some have specific legislation to protect health information. This latter development is, in part, a response to the public backlash to initial efforts to establish electronic health information networks and EHRs, including patient records. While privacy concerns about health records pre-dated such efforts, the potential use of EHRs has highlighted these concerns.

2.7.2 Health research

There are a handful of university-based research centres focused on health services and policy research including the MCHP, the Centre for Health Economics and Policy Analysis (CHEPA) at McMaster University, the Centre for Health Services and Policy Research (CHSPR) at the University of British Columbia, and IRSPUM (Institut de recherche en santé publique) at the University of Montreal.

Researchers are funded through national and provincial health funding organizations. The CIHR Institute of Health Services and Policy Research is the single largest health services and policy research institute in Canada, although other CIHR institutes, including those for Aboriginal People's Health, Gender and Health and Population and Public Health, also invest in health services and policy research. An alliance of provincial health research funding agencies, the National Alliance of Provincial Health Research Organizations (NAPHRO), was created in 2003 to promote collaboration on common issues. Its members include:

- Michael Smith Foundation for Health Research (BC)
- Alberta Innovates – Health Solutions
- Saskatchewan Health Research Foundation
- Manitoba Health Research Council
- Ontario Ministry of Health and Long-Term Care
- Ontario Ministry of Research and Innovation
- Fonds de la recherche en santé du Québec
- New Brunswick Health Research Foundation
- Nova Scotia Health Research Foundation
- Newfoundland and Labrador Centre for Applied Health Research.

2.7.3 Health technology assessment

Objective and reliable HTA is essential for effective planning as well as for evidence-based decision-making by health managers and providers. Most technological progress is incremental, and new advances tend to build directly on existing ideas, products and techniques, but some technological change involves major breakthroughs in terms of new products (e.g. new cancer drugs) or new techniques (e.g. bariatric surgery). An often used example of the latter involves genetic testing and gene technologies and HTA agencies must deal with both types of technological change (Giacomini, Miller & Browman, 2003; Morgan & Hurley, 2004; Rogowski, 2007). While HTA reports that include an economic evaluation are useful to health system decision-makers operating under a budget constraint, they involve more time and expense to complete than HTAs, which only address clinical effectiveness. Tarride et al. (2008) found that less than 25% of HTAs in Canada included an economic evaluation although it is unclear how this compares with HTA agencies outside Canada.

HTA organizations operate at provincial and at the pan-Canadian levels. Currently, there are three provincial HTA agencies. The first fully fledged HTA agency, the Agence d'évaluation de technologies et des modes d'intervention en santé (AETMIS)[4], was established in Quebec in 1988. In 2011, AETMIS was renamed INESSS – l'Institut national d'excellence en santé et en services sociaux. The second is the Ontario Health Technology Advisory Committee and the Medical Advisory Secretariat, once part of the Ministry of Health and Long-Term Care, but now part of Health Quality Ontario, an arm's length public agency. The third provincially based organization is in Alberta, where the HTA unit at the Institute of Health Economics (IHE)[5] makes recommendations to Alberta Health Services and the provincial ministry of health (Hailey, 2007; Menon & Stafinski, 2009). In addition, there are numerous academic and hospital-based organizations that conduct HTAs (Battista et al., 2009).

The CADTH is the sole pan-Canadian HTA agency and it is also the largest producer of HTAs in the country. Established and funded by F/P/T governments, CADTH's mandate is to provide evidence-based evaluations of new health technologies including prescription drugs and medical devices, procedures and systems (see section 2.3.3) to all participating governments.[6] These recommendations are advisory in nature and it is up to the governments to decide whether or not to introduce medical technologies or add prescription drugs to their respective health systems and public drug plans (Hailey, 2007).

Established in 2003, CADTH's CDR streamlines the process for reviewing new pharmaceuticals and providing recommendations to all provinces and territories except Quebec. The CDR process has three stages: (1) CADTH does a systematic review of the clinical evidence and pharmaco-economic data; (2) the Canadian Expert Drug Advisory Committee (CEDAC) under

[4] AETMIS was originally incorporated as the Conseil d'évaluation des technologies de la santé, the name which it retained until renamed in 2000.

[5] Until 2006, the HTA unit at IHE was housed at the Alberta Heritage Foundation for Medical Research.

[6] All participating member governments have a seat on CADTH's board of directors. Quebec is not a founding member of CADTH and has no seat on the CADTH board (CADTH, 2011).

CADTH makes a formulary listing recommendation; and (3) health ministries make their own formulary and benefit coverage decisions on the basis of their own drug formulary committees, policy environments and political pressures. Provincial decisions can be influenced by the presence or absence of a significant pharmaceutical industry presence. In Canada, the majority of pharmaceutical production is concentrated in two cities – Toronto (Ontario) and Montreal (Quebec).

2.8 Regulation

While provincial governments have primary jurisdiction over the administration and delivery of public health care services, health ministries delegate actual delivery to physicians and individual health care organizations. Health facilities and organizations – from independent hospitals and long-term care establishments to RHAs – are regulated by provincial governments. RHAs are delegated authorities rather than governments and as such have no law-making capacity. As a consequence, RHAs operate under provincial laws and regulations. The medical and financial coverage provided to employees under provincial and territorial WCBs are regulated by provincial and territorial governments.

Health organizations, including RHAs and independent health facilities, are accredited on a voluntary basis through Accreditation Canada, a member-based, non governmental organization. Most health care providers, including physicians, nurses, dentists, optometrists, chiropractors, physiotherapists, occupational therapists, are organized as self-governing professions under provincial and territorial law.

2.8.1 Regulation and governance of third-party payers

Provincial and territorial ministries of health are the principal third-party payers in Canada. All these governments administer their own single-payer medicare coverage systems under their own laws and regulations (see section 9.3.2). As the principal payers, provincial ministries and RHAs work through, and contract with, a range of independent health care organizations including hospitals, day surgeries, diagnostic clinics, medical laboratories, emergency transportation companies, long-term care organizations and primary health clinics. Although this institutional arrangement appears similar to the internal market in the United Kingdom, it does not imply the same purchaser–provider arrangements as in the National Health Service (Boyle, 2011).

In the provinces that are currently regionalized, provincial governments have laws that define, in very high-level directional terms, the division of responsibility and accountability between their respective ministries of health and RHAs. Some RHAs, such as the local health integrated networks in Ontario, are subject to targets based on performance measures. However, provincial ministers of health and provincial governments remain ultimately accountable to their residents for ensuring access to, as well as the timeliness and quality of, public health care goods and services.

Although a similar accountability relationship exists in Canada's three territories, these jurisdictions are constitutionally and fiscally dependent on the federal government. As such, they have been delegated the responsibility and accountability for the administration of public health care services as well as providing first-dollar coverage for medically necessary hospital and physician services. However, as a consequence of the territories having an inadequate tax base to fund such services – combined with the much higher cost of delivering services in the sparsely populated north – territorial governments are heavily reliant on federal fiscal transfers well beyond their per capita allocation under the Canada Health Transfer (Young & Chatwood, 2011; Marchildon & Chatwood, 2012).

As noted above, the federal government provides some non-medicare health services to registered members of First Nation communities as well as eligible Inuit. In recent decades, this responsibility has been turned over to some indigenous communities through self-governing agreements (Minore & Katt, 2007). However, it is the Government of Canada's position that the health programmes, services and insurance coverage it provides to First Nation and Inuit beneficiaries is on the basis of national policy and not due to any constitutional or Aboriginal treaty obligations, a position contested by a majority of First Nation and Inuit governments and organizations.

While there is an active market for PHI that is either complementary or supplementary to medicare, PHI for medicare services is either prohibited or discouraged by provincial and territorial laws, regulations and long-established policy practices (Flood & Archibald, 2001) (see section 3.6). Both the federal and provincial governments are involved in regulating PHI, the vast majority of which comes in the form of group insurance plans sponsored by employers, in which individual beneficiaries have limited or no choice of insurer (Hurley & Guindon, 2008; Gechert, 2010). The federal government is responsible for regulating the solvency of insurance carriers, while the provincial and territorial governments are responsible for regulating the actual insurance product, including the design and pricing of the health coverage package as well as consumer sale and service.

2.8.2 Regulation and governance of providers

Providers can be either organizations, such as RHAs, hospitals, long-term care homes and medical clinics, or individual health professionals. Historically, the vast majority of hospitals in Canada have been private, mainly non-profit-making, institutions that operated at arm's length from provincial governments, although some government regulation and supervision had long been accepted by those hospitals accepting subsidies for indigent patients. However, with the introduction of universal hospital coverage throughout Canada, the relationship between hospitals and provincial governments became much closer, with hospitals almost entirely reliant on public funding and governments ultimately accountable for the use of public funds. With regionalization, hospitals have been drawn into an even tighter relationship with provincial governments. Indeed, in many provinces, the majority of hospitals are now owned and operated by the RHAs, and the remaining independent hospitals are contractually obliged to provide RHA residents with acute care services (Maddelena, 2006; Philippon & Braithwaite, 2008). Except for Alberta and Quebec, accreditation remains voluntary and nongovernmental in nature and is performed in all jurisdictions by Accreditation Canada (see section 2.3.4).

Redress for medical malpractice and similar negligence based on the common law of tort is pursued privately through the courts.[7] Both physicians (as independent contractors as opposed to employees) and health organizations (who are responsible for the quality and safety of the service delivered by their salaried providers) can be sued. There is considerable debate concerning the benefits of such lawsuits in terms of improving the standard and quality of care. Moreover, there is some evidence that the incentives created by the private tort system can potentially impede health care reform, especially the establishment and effective functioning of multi professional primary health care teams, by continuing to hold physicians accountable for any alleged malpractice committed by a non-physician member of the team (Mohr, 2000; Caulfield, 2004) (complaints procedures available to patients are described in section 2.9.4).

[7] In contrast to other provinces in Canada, Quebec has a civil code rather than common law, and medical malpractice is governed under the provision regarding general civil liability under its civil code.

Damage awards and, therefore, malpractice insurance costs are lower in Canada than the United States for a number of reasons, including the more restricted practice of contingency billing by lawyers; the lower damages awarded by Canadian courts, in which judges rather than juries assess the quantum of damages; and the policy of physician associations to fight rather than settle "nuisance" claims (Mohr, 2000). Unfortunately, these differences have not produced an environment in which Canadian physicians are more prepared than their American colleagues to report medical errors to patients (Levinson & Gallagher, 2007).

There has been no major empirical study and reassessment of medical malpractice in Canada since the Prichard study commissioned by F/P/T deputy ministers of health in the late 1980s (Prichard, 1990). Despite the serious problems associated with the private tort system, the Prichard Report nonetheless rejected the policy alternative of governments moving to a no-fault compensation system, and medical malpractice remains in place in every province and territory.

There are three different approaches taken by provinces and territories to provider regulation in Canada. The first approach – licensure – grants members of a profession (e.g. doctors and RNs) the exclusive right to provide a particular service to the public. The second – certification – allows both members and non-members of a profession (e.g. psychologists) to provide services to the public, but only certified or registered members can use the professional designation. The third approach – the controlled acts system – regulates a specific task or activity.

While the specific regulatory approach for provider groups can vary considerably across provinces and territories, there is remarkable consistency in approach among certain professions such as physicians, nurses and dentists across all jurisdictions. Moreover, there have been considerable intergovernmental efforts to address the issue of portability of qualifications among provinces due to each registered health profession having its own rules concerning the registration of its members within a province or territory. The self-regulated professions are expected to ensure that members are properly educated and trained and to enforce minimal quality of care standards.

In some provinces (British Columbia, Alberta, Saskatchewan, Ontario, Quebec, and New Brunswick), governments have also established health quality councils to work with the health professionals and health care organizations to improve quality standards and outcomes as well as report quality outcomes to the general public. However, none of these organizations has a mandate to enforce, much less regulate, quality standards. Although interprofessional care has become a desired objective among governments, health care organizations and provider groups, there remain a number of barriers to implementation, including segregated education and training and institutional arrangements concerning remuneration and malpractice (Lahey & Currie, 2005; HPRAC, 2008).

2.8.3 Registration and planning of human resources

Due to provincial jurisdiction over health human resources, there is no single, national system of registration and planning of human resources in Canada (Wranik, 2008). The RCPSC, for example, is not a licensing body even though it sets standards for specialist medical education in Canada and is responsible for certifying specialists. Physicians certified by the RCPSC are not required to be registered as members of the RCPSC. While the Health Council of Canada provides high-level analyses of health human resource issues at a pan-Canadian level, P/T governments are ultimately responsible for the regulation of the professions and human resource planning.

In an effort to facilitate greater collaboration on a pan-Canadian basis, the F/P/T Conference of Deputy Ministers of Health created the Advisory Committee on Health Delivery and Human Resources (ACHDHR) in 2002. In 2005, the ACHDHR created a framework with the following three key objectives, subsequently endorsed by F/P/T ministers of health (ACHDHR, 2007; Dumont et al., 2008):

- avoid the risks and duplication associated with the current jurisdiction-by-jurisdiction approach to human resources planning;
- overcome barriers to implementing system design including population needs-based planning; and
- increase health workforce planning capacity.

In response to concerns about how best to pursue health workforce self-sufficiency in response to both the perception and the reality of shortages in all jurisdictions, the ACHDHR also conducted a human resource study on behalf of F/P/T governments (ACHDHR, 2009). To date, there has been no major evaluation conducted on the changes precipitated by ACHDHR's initiatives.

Ontario's ministry of health has been among the most active governments in Canada in using regulation as a tool in human resource policy and planning (O'Reilly, 2000). This has included the introduction of a single law that provides a common regulatory framework for all the health professions and the establishment of a permanent Health Professions Regulatory Advisory Council (HPRAC) in the 1990s. The goals of the law include promoting higher quality care, treating professionals equitably by providing a single set of regulatory principles, improving the accountability of the professions to patients and providing more choice by ensuring access to a range of providers. In its 2006 report, HPRAC recommended a number of changes to the 21 regulatory colleges governing 23 health professions under Ontario's Regulated Health Professions Act to facilitate more effective human resource policy and planning. For example, HPRAC recommended that new stand-alone colleges with the powers of self-regulation be created for psychotherapists, kinesiologists, naturopaths and homeopaths, and that optometrists be granted authority to prescribe pharmaceutical therapies (HPRAC, 2006).

2.8.4 Regulation and governance of pharmaceuticals and natural health products

Only physicians are legally permitted to prescribe a full range of pharmaceutical therapies. However, in recent years, a number of provincial governments have changed their laws and regulations in order to permit some providers, including nurse practitioners, pharmacists and dentists, to have limited authority to prescribe pharmaceutical therapies within their respective scopes of practice.

Through its Therapeutic Products Directorate and the Biologics and Genetics Therapies Directorate, Health Canada determines the initial approval and labelling of all prescription drugs. In 2004, the Natural Health Products Directorate was established, and Health Canada began to regulate traditional herbal medicines, vitamins and mineral supplements as well as homeopathic preparations in terms of initial approval and labelling. Health Canada also prohibits direct-to-consumer advertising (DTCA) of prescription drug products, a prohibition that has been challenged as contrary to the Charter of Rights and Freedoms by one of Canada's largest media chains (Flood, 2010). Despite the current prohibition, a large proportion of the Canadian public is influenced by DTCA through cable and satellite television networks that originate in the United States where DTCA is permitted. Advertising of prescription drugs to health professionals is subject to federal legislation as well as to advertising and ethical practices codes established by industry associations (Mintzes et al., 2002; Paris & Docteur, 2006).

The constitution confers exclusive jurisdiction over the patenting of new inventions, including novel prescription drugs, to the federal government. The Patent Office is part of the Canadian Intellectual Property Office, a special operating agency associated with the Federal Department of Industry Canada. In the late 1980s and early 1990s, the federal government shifted policy direction by increasing patent protection to the OECD norm of 20 years and by abolishing compulsory licensing in an effort to increase the level of investment, research and development by the international pharmaceutical industry in Canada (Anis, 2000). At the same time, the federal government established the PMPRB to regulate the factory gate prices of patented drugs (see section 2.3.2). Provincial and territorial governments use a number of regulatory tools to contain the cost of their respective drug plans although these vary considerably across jurisdictions. These regulatory tools include reference pricing (reimbursing on the basis of the lowest cost pharmaceutical in a given therapeutic category), licensing, bulk purchasing, tendering and discounting (Paris & Docteur, 2006; Grootendorst & Hollis, 2011).

2.8.5 Regulation of medical devices and aids

The federal government regulates medical devices through the Medical Devices Program in the Therapeutic Products Division of Health Canada. Diagnostic and therapeutic medical devices fall under one of the four enumerated classes in the Medical Devices Regulations of the federal Food and Drugs Act (see Table 2.4). The Medical Devices Program assesses the safety, effectiveness and quality of medical devices by a combination of pre-market review, post-approval surveillance and quality systems in the manufacturing process (Health Canada, 2007).

Canada is also an active participant in the International Medical Device Regulators' Forum, which is working towards harmonizing the regulation for medical devices in all participating countries. Health Canada is also engaged in two bilateral harmonization initiatives, one with the Food and Drug Administration in the United States to develop, manage and oversee a new process that will allow a single regulatory audit to satisfy the needs of multiple regulatory jurisdictions, and the second with the Therapeutic Goods Administration in Australia to mutually recognize Quality Management Systems certification for medical device manufacturers (Health Canada, 2007).

Table 2.4
Health Canada's medical device classification under the Food and Drugs Act

Device class	Risk	Examples	Licence requirements
I	Lowest	Reusable surgical instruments, bandages and laboratory culture media	Device licence not required but establishment where device is made or distributed must be licensed
II	Low	Contact lenses, pregnancy test kits, endoscopes, catheters	Manufacturers require a Health Canada licence before selling or advertising medical devices. Manufacturers are also required to renew licence annually
III	Moderate	Orthopaedic implants, glucose monitors, dental implants, haemodialysis machines	
IV	High	Cardiac pacemakers, angiogram catheters, cranial shunts	

Source: Health Canada (2007).

2.8.6 Regulation of capital investment

In contrast to the federal regulation of medical devices, capital investments in health care are regulated at the provincial level. In most cases, formal laws and regulation do not exist. Instead, P/T governments make an annual decision on capital projects through the budget process. Similarly, RHAs also make decisions based on their own annual budgets although P/T ministries of health make major capital investment decisions, such as new hospital construction. Independent hospitals make their own capital investment decisions but those that have contracts with RHAs will work in tandem with the RHAs on major capital expansions. Private health care organizations delivering non-medicare services, including long-term care, rehabilitation, dental and vision care services, are generally free to make their own capital investment decisions without regulatory oversight.

In the 1990s, some provincial governments, such as Alberta and Saskatchewan, enacted laws to regulate the establishment and expansion of private facilities providing acute care services including surgery clinics (McIntosh & Ducie, 2009). Despite the rapid growth in private surgery clinics, most provincial governments have been slow to introduce comprehensive regulation and monitoring (Lett, 2008; Glauser, 2011).

2.9 Patient empowerment

2.9.1 Patient information

Most patients in Canada rely heavily on information provided by their health care providers, in particular their family physicians as well as the specialist physicians to whom they are referred. This information and advice is supplemented by information provided by health care organizations, including hospitals, RHAs and province-wide programmes, particularly for the prevention, diagnosis and treatment of cancer. In the case of cancer, almost all provinces have patient navigation programmes. In some provinces, such as Nova Scotia and Quebec, cancer care navigators, most of whom are nurses, must have a minimal level of experience to be certified (Wackinshaw, 2011; Pederson & Hack, 2011).

The Canadian Council on Literacy defines health literacy as the ability to obtain, understand and use health information. According to Simach (2009), health literacy is a strong predictor of health status. Based on an International Adult Literacy and Skills Survey of 23 000 Canadians using the Health Activities Literacy Scale, which assesses literacy in terms of health promotion, health protection, disease prevention, health care maintenance and system navigation, roughly 60% of Canadians lack the capacity to obtain, understand and act on health information and services to make appropriate health decisions (Canadian Council on Learning, 2007). Immigrants, particularly those who come from countries where the cultures and health systems differ greatly from those in Canada, as well as new immigrants whose first language is neither English nor French, have even lower health literacy than the already low Canadian mean (Ng & Omariba, 2010).

There is a modest amount of accessible information on the quality of health services in Canada. Since its creation in 2003, the Health Council of Canada (HCC) has produced a number of reports, videos, podcasts and electronic newsletters aimed at the general public. The HCC has also focused on issues of patient and citizen engagement, including the engagement of Canadians in their own primary health care (HCC, 2011b). Although provincial health quality councils were established mainly to provide health ministries and RHAs with systematic advice on quality improvement, they have also served to inform the public on key aspects of health care. In recent years, provincial ministries, quality councils and other organizations have provided more information to the public on issues of great public interest including surgical waiting times and hospital report cards. Historically, Canadians received little direct information on medical errors, and critical incidents; however, the Canadian Patient Safety Institute has led a major initiative to produce guidelines for the disclosure of medical errors, with a revised version released in 2011 (CPSI, 2008, 2011), while other researchers associated with major health care agencies in Canada have suggested disclosure guidelines in situations where a given error affects numerous patients (Chafe, Levinson & Sullivan, 2009).

A number of provincial governments have issued general statements and booklets concerning the public health care benefits to which residents are entitled. These statements are generally available on ministry of health websites. Similarly, the federal government has used its departmental websites to provide information on the health benefits provided to (for example) eligible First Nations, Inuit and veterans.

2.9.2 Patient choice

Within the limits imposed by geographical distance and isolation, provincial and territorial residents are at liberty to choose the physician, hospital or long-term care facility. Even residents living within a particular RHA can choose to access the services of a facility in another RHA in the same province. However, other than in an emergency, they cannot obtain insured medicare services in another province or country without a prior referral by an eligible authority in their own province.

In the last 15 years, a patient's choice of primary care provider has been constrained by the supply of family physicians in some locations as well as the desire by some physicians to limit their roster to potentially less demanding patients (Asanin & Wilson, 2008; Reid et al., 2009). Since family physicians act as gatekeepers in most provinces, patients are prevented or discouraged from approaching consulting physicians directly. However, at the point of referral, Canadians do have a choice of specialist.

2.9.3 Patient rights

Two royal commission reports, one in 1964 and a second in 2002, have recommended a pan-Canadian patient charter of rights (Canada, 1964; Romanow, 2002). Despite this, there is no national patient charter of rights in Canada. In addition, no province or territory has implemented a patient charter of rights or other laws defining specific individual patient rights (Smith, 2002).

The patient rights movement is relatively underdeveloped in Canada, at least compared with similar movements in the United States and Western Europe. While there are organizations (e.g. Canadian Cancer Society and the Canadian Mental Health Association) that advocate for the rights of patients with particular diseases, there are only a few individually oriented patient rights groups and these tend to be very weak in comparison with the specific disease-oriented organizations (Golding, 2005). While more general purpose organizations such as the Consumers' Association of Canada and the Canadian Association of Retired Persons have engaged in some patient advocacy, these efforts remain limited compared with individually oriented patient rights organizations in other countries.

Historically, individual patient rights in Canada have largely been defined in terms of a perceived "right" of access to universally insured medicare services under the Canada Health Act. Since the introduction of the Charter of Rights and Freedoms in 1982, there have been a small number of cases in which patients have challenged provincial governments' interpretation of what the basket of universal health services includes. In addition, the question has arisen whether section 7, the "right to life, liberty and security of the person", of the Charter of Rights and Freedoms encompasses a right of access to health care within a reasonable time (Greschner, 2004; Jackman, 2004). Thus far, the Supreme Court of Canada has not interpreted section 7 to include such a right (Flood, Roach & Sossin, 2005; Flood, 2007). Indeed, while it appears that the Supreme Court is concerned about provincial restrictions on private insurance for medicare services and is prepared to extend the right to private health services as demonstrated in the Chaoulli decision of 2005, it has not yet been willing to use the Charter to extend or enhance current rights to publicly financed medicare services (Cousin, 2009).

All F/P/T governments have general laws to ensure that disabled residents have access to public facilities or to facilities that serve the general public. Since virtually all health care facilities come within this definition, disabled persons are ensured physical access to health services.

2.9.4 Complaints procedures (mediation, claims)

Historically, concerns about public health care were either expressed to provincial and territorial ministries of health and their ministers or to members of opposition parties, who would then question the governing party through the media and in the legislature. It is likely that only a tiny minority of patients ever used this highly political procedure and there has been growing pressure on governments to establish less difficult complaints procedures. As a consequence, some provincial and territorial ministries of health (through external ombudsmen offices or a ministry office), RHAs and hospitals have established internal complaints procedures, although the main remedy remains private – through complaints to private professional regulatory authorities at the provincial and territorial level of government. These complaints can range from concerns about the poor bed manners of some health professionals at one end of the spectrum to allegations of life-threatening medical errors (for a discussion of the possibility of obtaining redress through the tort system, see section 2.8.2).

2.9.5 Public participation, patient satisfaction and patient-centred care

Other than through general participation in the political system, there are few formal vehicles for direct public participation in health system decision-making. At the time regionalization was introduced in Canada, one of the stated objectives was to extend public participation through elected RHA boards. For the most part, this objective was either not implemented or, when implemented in a few jurisdictions, was altered subsequently (Lewis & Kouri, 2004; Chessie, 2009). Today, the majority of RHA board members are appointed by provincial ministers or ministries of health and participation is largely limited to input from self-selected or appointed citizen advisory groups (Chessie, 2010).

Based on the results of recent Commonwealth Fund surveys of all patients (HCC 2010b) and sicker patients (Schoen et al., 2011) in 11 high-income countries, Canadians expressed considerable dissatisfaction about numerous aspects of provider access and the quality of the services they received (Table 2.5). In the more general 2010 survey, Canadians had among the poorest outcomes in terms of access to a doctor or nurse, waiting times for elective surgery or to see a specialist, and the highest reliance on emergency departments for care (Schoen, Osborn & Squires, 2010). Consequently, 61% of the patients sampled felt that the Canadian health system was in need of fundamental reforms or to be rebuilt completely, which was lower than in Australia (75%) and the United States (68%) but higher than France (58%), Sweden (53%) and the United Kingdom (37%). However, the 2011 survey results for sicker patients reflect better-than-average results in terms of health system coordination and shared decision-making with specialist physicians.

Table 2.5
Survey of sicker adults in terms of access, coordination and patient-centred experience, 2011 (% of patients)

	Access to doctor or nurse when sick or in need of care								
	Same day or next day appointment	Waited 6 days or more	Difficulty getting after-hours care without going to ED	Used emergency department in past 2 years	Waited less than 1 month to see a specialist	Experienced coordination gaps in past 2 years	Experienced gaps in hospital or surgery discharge in past 2 years	Any medical, medication or laboratory errors in past 2 years	Shared decision-making with specialist
Australia	63	10	56	48	59	36	55	19	64
Canada	51	23	63	58	52	40	50	21	61
France	75	8	55	33	67	53	73	13	37
Sweden	50	22	52	50	63	39	67	20	48
United Kingdom	79	2	21	40	80	20	26	8	79
United States	59	16	55	49	88	42	29	22	67

Source: Derived from Schoen et al. (2011).
Note: ED: Emergency department.

Since 2008, some provincial ministries of health have launched patient-centred care initiatives. In Saskatchewan, for example, an externally appointed ministerial advisory committee, known as the Patient First Review, consulted patients and caregivers and reviewed existing care processes before making a series of recommendations for change (Dagnone, 2009). In Ontario, the provincial government passed a law entitled "Excellent Care for All" that requires hospitals to engage with their patients and caregivers in order to gauge the level of satisfaction with services, and requires health care organizations to develop a declaration of values based in public input.

2.9.6 Patients and cross-border health

Under the portability provision of the Canada Health Act, provincial and territorial governments are required to provide coverage for insured hospital and physician services for their residents when they are visiting other jurisdictions, both inside and outside Canada. Within Canada, section 11 of the Act requires that residents visiting other jurisdictions be reimbursed at the rate approved by the P/T plan in which the services are provided unless there is an agreement between the jurisdictions to do otherwise. Outside Canada, P/T plans are to reimburse the amount that would have been paid in the home province or territory.

Provinces and territories are allowed to require patients to get consent from their home jurisdiction before seeking elective (non-emergency) medicare services in another province or country. Within Canada, the portability provisions of the Canada Health Act are implemented through a series of bilateral billing agreements between the provinces and territories for hospital and physician services. All provinces and territories participate in hospital reciprocal billing and all, with the exception of Quebec, participate in reciprocal medical agreements. To date, the federal government has chosen not to enforce this breach of the portability condition (Flood & Choudhry, 2004).

3. Financing

The public sector in Canada is responsible for almost 70% of total health expenditures (THE). After a period of spending restraint in the early to mid-1990s, government expenditures have grown rapidly, at a rate of growth only exceeded by private health expenditure. Since health expenditures have grown more rapidly than either the growth in the economy or public revenues, this growth has triggered concerns about the fiscal sustainability of public health care. Contrary to popular perception, demographic ageing has not, at least yet, been a major driver of health system costs in Canada. Over the last two decades, prescription drugs have been a major cost driver, but in the last five years, the growth in this sector has been matched by hospital spending and overtaken by physician expenditures. In the case of physicians, a primary cost driver has been increased remuneration, and in the case of hospitals, a combination of more hiring and increased remuneration for existing staff (CIHI, 2011b).

Almost all revenues for public health spending come from the general tax revenues of F/P/T governments, a considerable portion of which is used to provide universal medicare – medically necessary hospital and physician services that are free at the point of service. The remaining amount is used to subsidize other types of health care, including long-term care and prescription drugs. While the provinces raise the majority of funds through own-source revenues, they also receive less than a quarter of their health financing from the Canada Health Transfer, an annual cash transfer from the federal government. On the private side, OOP payments and PHI are responsible for most health revenues. The vast majority of PHI comes in the form of compulsory employment-based insurance for non-medicare goods and services including prescription drugs, dental care and vision care. PHI does not compete with the provincial and territorial "single payer" systems for medicare.

3.1 Health expenditure

Of the total of C$200 billion spent on health care in 2011, almost 43% was directed to hospital and physician services. If medically necessary, these services are defined as "insured services" under the Canada Health Act. Almost 30% was spent on private health care services, a large proportion of which was for dental and vision care services as well as over-the-counter pharmaceuticals and privately paid prescription drugs. An additional 23.5% was spent by governments on health infrastructure and publicly funded or subsidized non-medicare services. Finally, 3.5% was devoted to direct federal services including benefits for special populations such as First Nations living on reserves and Inuit residing in northern land claim regions, as well as health research and the regulation of medicines (CIHI, 2010b).

Table 3.1
Trends in health expenditure in Canada, 1995–2010 (selected years)

	1995	2000	2005	2010
THE $US PPP per capita	2 054.1	2 518.9	3 441.9	4 478.2
THE as % of GDP	9.0	8.8	9.8	11.3
Public health expenditure as % of GDP	6.4	6.2	6.9	8.0
Public health expenditure as % of THE	71.2	70.4	70.2	70.5
Private expenditure on health as % of THE	28.8	29.6	29.8	29.5
Private expenditure on health as % of total government spending	40.4	42.1	42.4	41.9
OOP payments as % of THE	15.9	15.9	14.6	14.7
OOP payments as % of private expenditure on health	55.2	53.7	49.1	49.7
PHI as % of THE	10.3	11.5	12.6	12.8
PHI as % of private expenditure on health	35.8	38.8	42.3	43.3

Source: Calculated based on OECD (2011a).
Note: THE, total health expenditure; OOP, out-of-pocket; PHI, private health insurance.

As shown in Table 3.1, Canada has experienced rapid growth in THE in recent years, whether measured by per capita increases in spending or as a percentage of economic growth. Real annual growth in THE reached a peak in the late 1970s and the early 1980s, then declined precipitously in the early to mid-1990s only to rise again by the end of the 20th century. From the early 1990s until 1997, health expenditure growth, particularly public sector health expenditure growth, was substantially below GDP growth as a consequence of major funding constraints by provincial health ministries, producing a real (inflation-adjusted) decline in public health care spending (Tuohy, 2002). Throughout this period of public restraint, the growth in private health spending outstripped public health spending. By the end of the 1990s, provincial governments had increased spending on health care. By 2000, the federal government had begun to increase cash transfers to the provinces that culminated with a commitment in 2004 to apply an automatic rate of annual increase of 6% for the following 10 years (CICS, 2004).

Although both public and private spending per capita has increased since 1995, private-sector health expenditures have grown more rapidly than government spending. This is partially a result of technological developments that have allowed fully covered inpatient services to be shifted to outpatient settings with less complete public coverage. Canada's share of private health expenditures, in part the product of almost no public coverage for dental care and vision care, is high by other OECD country standards (CIHI 2011a).

As can be seen in Figs 3.1 and 3.2, Canada's recent experience in terms of the growth of health spending as a share of the economy is similar to other OECD countries. The one exception is the United States, which spends appreciably more as a proportion of its economy.

Fig. 3.1

Trends in total health expenditure as a share of GDP in Canada and selected countries, 1990–2010

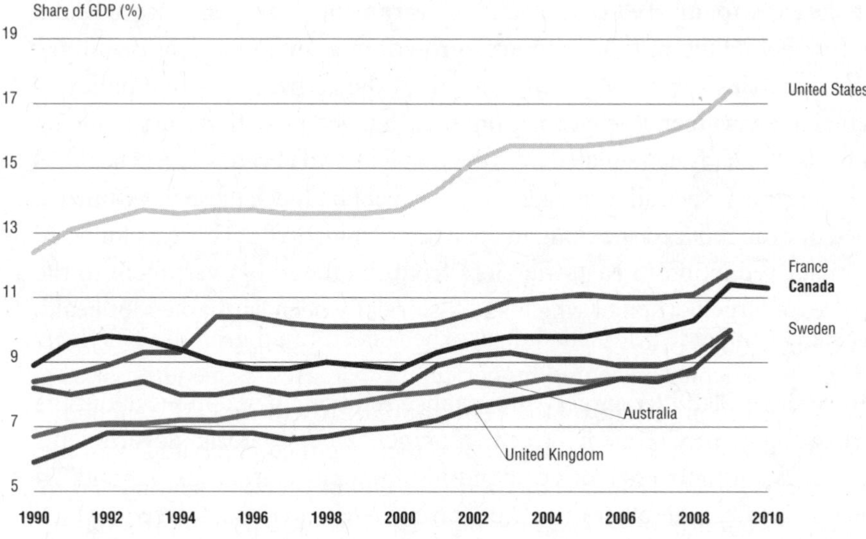

Source: OECD (2011).
Note: 2010 data was available only for Canada, not for other countries.

Fig. 3.2
Trends in total health expenditure per capita ($US PPP) in Canada and selected countries, 1990–2010

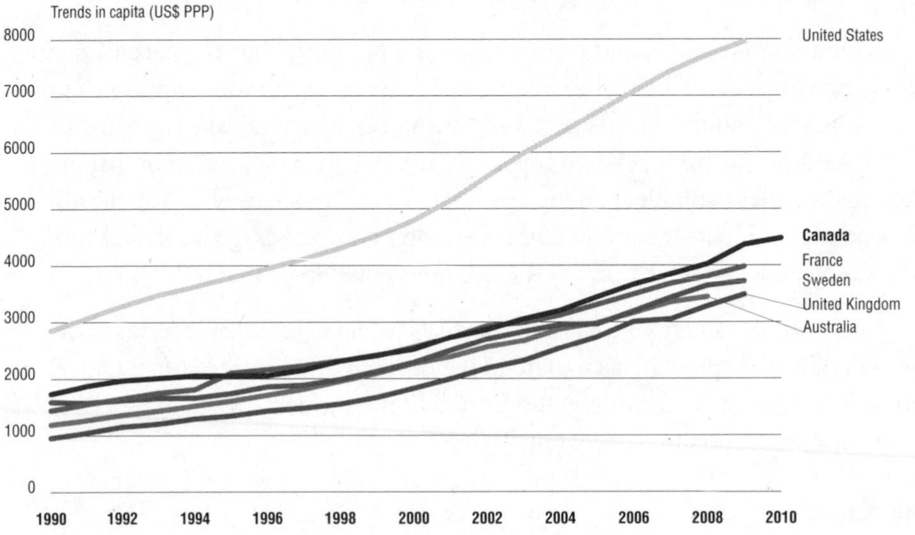

Source: OECD (2011).
Note: 2010 data was available only for Canada, not for other countries.

In the early to mid-1990s, Canadian Governments managed to force health spending below the rate of economic growth to a greater extent than most OECD countries. This was a direct result of the aggressive fiscal policy of provincial governments in eliminating their budgetary deficits and reducing debt loads that had accumulated over the previous two decades. Since health is the single largest spending category in provincial budgets, these governments capped or even reduced spending in the early to mid-1990s. This was followed by a major reduction in cash transfers from the federal government to the provinces, a large portion of which had historically been earmarked for health care (Tuohy, 2002).

Since the mid-1990s, largely in response to public perceptions about the deteriorating quality of medicare, the provincial and territorial governments have increased their respective spending on health care. Figs 3.3 and 3.4 compare Canada with other OECD countries in terms of the degree to which public-sector health spending has increased since 1990. While all six countries have shown considerable growth in public-sector health spending over the past 20 years whether measured as a share of the economy or in per capita terms, the latter measure demonstrates the extent to which the Canadian experience with respect to public expenditure has been almost identical to France, Sweden and the United Kingdom.

Fig. 3.3
Trends in public expenditure on health as a share of GDP in Canada and selected countries, 1990–2010

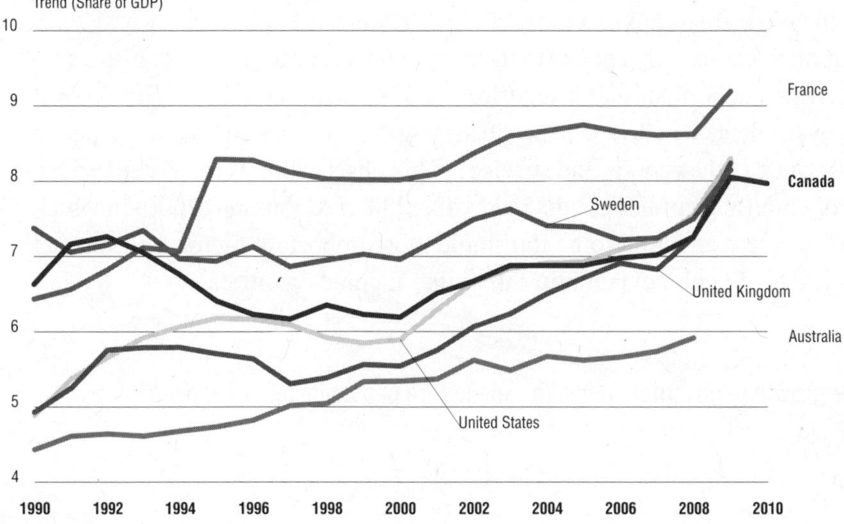

Source: OECD (2011).
Note: 2010 data was available only for Canada, not for other countries.

Fig. 3.4
Trends in public expenditure on health per capita ($US PPP) in Canada and selected countries, 1990–2010

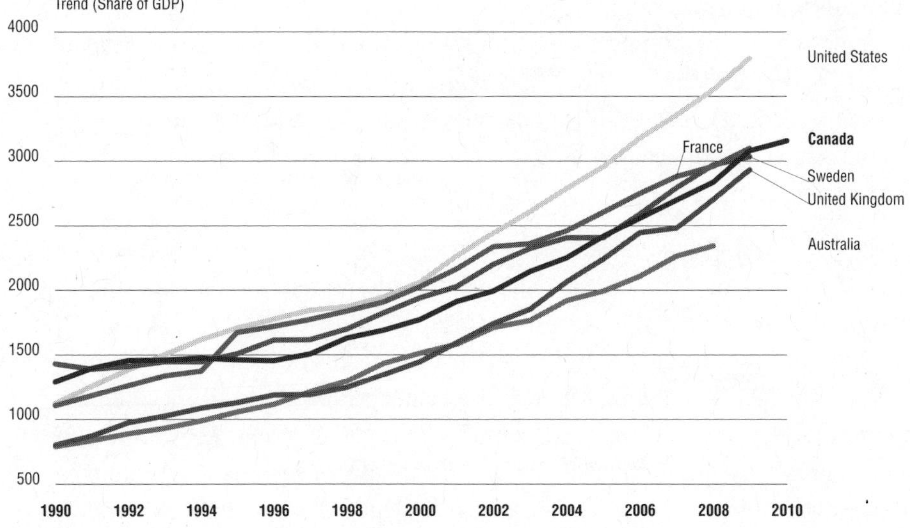

Source: OECD (2011).
Note: 2010 data was available only for Canada, not for other countries.

To gain a fuller appreciation of the link between economic growth and health spending, it is worthwhile comparing the Canadian experience with all higher income OECD countries for which comparable data are available. As can be seen in Fig. 3.5, total health spending exceeded economic growth (location above the 45 degree line) in almost all these countries between 1998 and 2008. Overall, this relationship speaks to the fact that health care is, to a considerable extent, what economists call a superior good. As national incomes go up over time, governments tend to spend progressively more of these increases on health care relative to other goods and services. This observation is consistent with a series of empirical studies conducted by Gerdtham & Jönsson (2000) in which higher income was found to be the single most important factor determining higher levels of health expenditure in higher income countries.

Fig. 3.5

Average growth in government health expenditure per capita and GDP per capita, 1998–2008

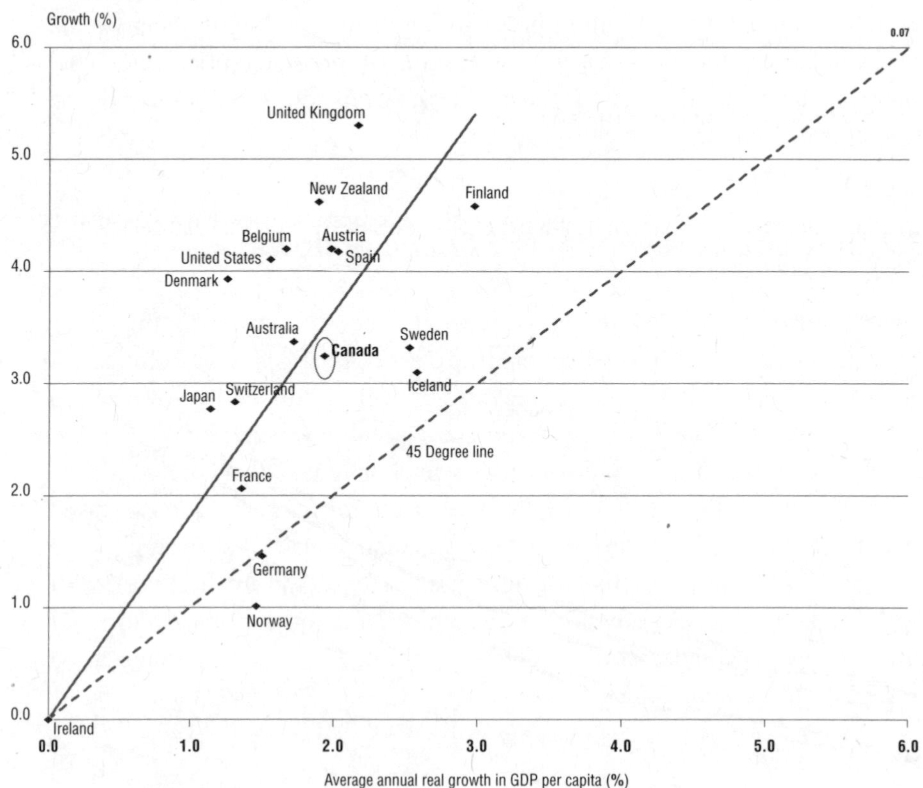

Source: CIHI (2011b).

To understand the underlying health cost drivers, it is essential to separate health spending by service programmes or functions, and then examine the impact of health-specific inflation, increased utilization and ageing. From the 1980s until the mid-2000s, prescription drugs were the fastest growing category of health expenditure, and most of this growth was due to a combination of increased utilization, the introduction of new drug therapies and higher prices. In this respect, Canada has had among the highest generic drug prices in the world (perhaps in part due to the lack of generic price regulation at the national level). In contrast, factory gate prices of branded prescription drug are regulated by the PMPRB while CADTH provides provincial governments with a centralized drug assessment and review process for new prescription drugs (Romanow, 2002; McMahon, Morgan & Mitton, 2006).

Since 2005, there has been an acceleration in spending on physicians driven more by increases in remuneration than volume. Hospital expenditures have also grown rapidly due mainly to increases in staffing levels, compensation and the increased use of advanced technologies, including advanced diagnostics. In sharp contrast, the growth in prescription drug spending in recent years has been largely due to increases in utilization as opposed to price, due to the maturing of patents as well as a slowing in the rate of new drugs coming on the market relative to previous periods (CIHI, 2011b).

3.2 Sources of revenue and financial flows

The principal source of health system finance is taxation by the F/T/P governments (see Fig. 3.6). Since medicare services are exempt from patient payment at the point of service, they are entirely financed by government revenues mainly at the provincial level. The sources of funding for other health goods and services are derived from a combination of taxation, OOP payments and PHI. The vast majority of PHI comes in the form of employment-based insurance that employees are required to take on as part of a given package of remuneration and benefits. Social insurance forms the smallest portion of health funding and is largely used for health benefits for workplace injuries or ailments available under workers' compensation schemes in the provinces and territories (see section 3.3.2).

Fig. 3.6
Percentage of total expenditure on health by source of revenue, 2010

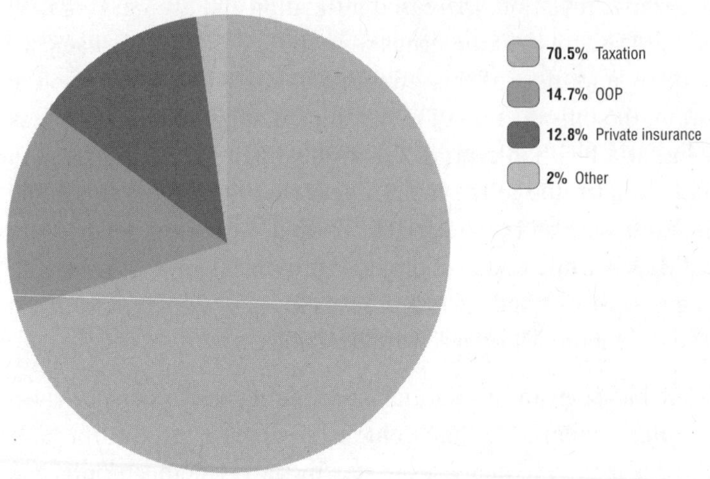

Source: OECD (2011a).

As can be seen in Table 3.2, which shows changes over time, the proportion of revenue from the four main sources changed only slightly between 1995 and 2009. General taxation has tended to provide well over two-thirds of all finance for health. PHI has grown more rapidly than OOP payments, in part because of the continuing centrality of PHI as part of employment-based benefit packages in unionized and professional workplaces.

Table 3.2
Sources of revenue as a percentage of total expenditure on health, 1995–2010 (selected years)

	1995	2000	2005	2006	2007	2008	2009	2010
General taxation	71.2	70.4	70.2	69.8	70.2	70.5	70.6	70.5
OOP	15.9	15.9	14.6	15.0	14.7	14.6	14.6	14.7
PHI	10.3	11.5	12.6	12.4	12.6	12.7	12.7	12.8
Social insurance funds	1.1	1.4	1.4	1.4	1.4	1.4	1.3	1.3

Source: OECD (2011a).

3.3 Overview of the statutory financing system

There are two levels of statutory or compulsory funding and coverage for health services. At the federal level, the Canada Health Act stipulates universal coverage for universally insured services administered at the provincial and territorial levels of government as a condition of providing fiscal transfers to support public insurance plans. At the provincial and territorial level, there are separate laws stipulating the right of access by residents, on the same terms and conditions, to medicare services (Fig. 3.7) (see section 9.3.2).

Fig. 3.7

Composition of financial flows in the Canadian health system

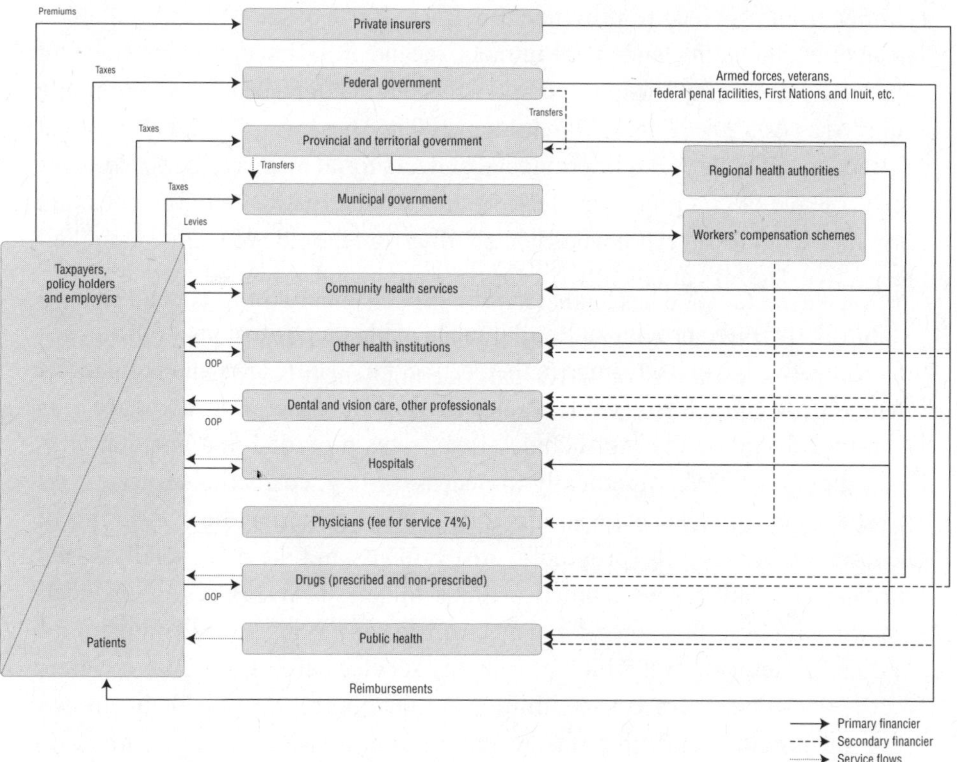

While the provinces and territories are most directly responsible for raising the majority of financing for publicly funded health care, the federal government contributes funding through transfers to these governments. The transfers to the Canada Health Transfer are conditional on the provinces and territories meeting the five conditions under the Canada Health Act (see section 2.3.2).

At the same time, some provinces receive unconditional transfers from the federal government through what is called equalization, while the territories receive unconditional transfers through another federal programme called Territorial Formula Financing. The specific purpose of equalization is to ensure that Canadians, wherever they live, "have access to reasonably comparable services at reasonably comparable levels of taxation", a purpose that is stated and protected in the Canadian Constitution (Expert Panel on Equalization and Territorial Formula Financing 2006, 18).

3.3.1 Coverage

The breadth, depth and scope of coverage for broadly defined insured services under the Canada Health Act (CHA), although not identical, are remarkably similar from province to province. In effect, 100% of the resident Canadian population, including landed immigrants, receive full (first dollar) coverage for "medically necessary" hospital, diagnostics and medical services, commonly summarized as "medicare" (Marchildon, 2009). These insured services are not defined in either the CHA or provincial and territorial medicare laws. However, the principle of comprehensiveness in the Canada Health Act presumes that provincial and territorial governments will err on the side of inclusion in their respective determinations of what services are included in medicare.

Similarly, at the provincial level, there is neither a positive list of inclusions nor a negative list of exclusions in the pertinent medicare laws and regulations. Instead, provincial governments have, from the time that medicare was first introduced, tended to include all services provided in a hospital with the exception of a few medically unnecessary (e.g. cosmetic) surgeries. As to which physician services are included, this has largely been a matter of negotiation between the provincial governments and the provincially based medical associations, but in practice almost all physician services are included. Ontario has one of the more formal mechanisms, involving three administrative bodies for determining which physicians services are universally covered: (1) the Physicians Services Committee, a joint committee of officials drawn from the provincial health ministry and the Ontario Medical Association; (2) Medical Directors – physicians employed by the provincial health ministry who determine claims for public funding; and (3) the provincial Health Services Appeal and Review Board (Flood, Stabile & Tuohy, 2006).

In terms of medicare, there has been no major reduction in, or expansion of, universally insured services by any level of government in Canada in recent years. Instead, most decisions involving new listings or delistings are highly marginal in nature and, in fact, most of them appear to address procedures beyond those required by medicare (Stabile & Ward, 2006). One historical exception involved the procedure to terminate pregnancy. After considerable debate and controversy, termination of pregnancy became an included medicare service in all jurisdictions except Prince Edward Island. Although clinical effectiveness is an important principle in decision-making concerning inclusion, HTA methods are not explicitly employed in these determinations.

Provincial and territorial governments administer medicare services through reimbursement schemes that prohibit or discourage supplementary private insurance (Flood & Archibald, 2001; Tuohy, 2009). Since provincial governments regulate the licensing of new facilities and work with provincial medical associations in regulating the billing of medicare, they have the capacity to limit or control the creation of a private (non-medicare) tier of hospitals, surgical clinics and physician services (McIntosh & Ducie, 2009). However, in some provinces, premium payments offered by workers' compensation schemes, in combination with the looser regulatory controls placed on diagnostic clinics and the desire by most provincial ministries of health to contract out to private medical laboratories have generated a market for private profit-making facilities (Hurley et al., 2008; Sutherland, 2011b).

Provincial governments receive compensation from the federal government for all medicare services provided to members of the Armed Forces, and inmates of federal prisons. Provincial and territorial governments must provide medicare services to all registered Indians and Inuit residents although the federal government provides these citizens with coverage for "non-insured health benefits" including dental care, prescription drug therapies and medical travel.

Beyond medicare, it is up to the provincial and territorial governments to decide the extent of coverage or subsidization for other health services. Since there is no pan-Canadian system or standards of coverage for non-medicare health services, it is very difficult to generalize concerning the breadth, depth and scope of coverage for non-medicare services, although there are at least three areas of convergence: (1) the majority of funding for long-term care is provided by the provinces and territories; (2) all jurisdictions provide pharmaceutical coverage for the older people and the very poor; and (3) virtually no public coverage is provided for dental care and vision or for CAM and therapies.

3.3.2 Collection

The dominant sources of funding are the general revenue funds of F/P/T governments. The bulk of provincial revenues is derived from individual income taxes, consumption taxes, corporation taxes and, at least in the case of resource-rich jurisdictions, resource royalties or taxes.

These general tax revenues are supplemented by health premiums in three provinces. In British Columbia, health premiums come in the form of a poll tax on individuals ($64 per year in 2012) and families ($116 for a family of two and $121 for a family of three or more in 2012), while in Ontario and Quebec they take the form of a surtax that is collected through a progressive income tax system.[1]

In both cases, premiums are only notionally earmarked for health spending and in fact flow into the general revenue funds of the provincial governments and thus are treated as part of general taxation. It should also be noted that health services cannot be denied on the basis of non-payment of premiums, and the provinces must rely on other remedies to enforce their collection. Health premiums raise less than 20% of what is expended by the provincial governments on health each year (McDonnell & McDonnell, 2005). A health premium in Alberta was eliminated in 2009, after a Task Force on Health Care Funding and Revenue Generation concluded that the premiums collected amounted to less than 13% of provincial health revenue needs (Alberta Health and wellness, 2002).

3.3.3 Pooling of funds and health system transfers

Budgetary allocations for health expenditures are made at three main levels in Canada: (1) the federal government (2) the provincial and territorial governments and (3) RHAs. At the federal and provincial levels, budgetary allocations are decided in cabinet and then reviewed and passed in the respective legislative chambers.

RHAs do not collect taxes but they allocate the funds they receive from ministries of health based on what they perceive to be the health demands of the populations they serve and the health care organizations and providers they fund. In the past, provincial RHA allocation formulas were used as a tool of health system reform – specifically to encourage more activity in upstream primary care and public health from downstream acute care. However, at least in most cases, these funding allocation formulas do not appear to have achieved

[1] At the time of writing, the government of Quebec announced its intention to repeal its health surtax.

their original reform objective (McIntosh et al., 2010). RHAs are required to submit their own draft budget to the ministry of health for approval. Some provincial governments explicitly forbid RHAs from running deficits, while others permit budget deficits under certain conditions (McKillop, 2004).

The Canada Health Transfer is the latest iteration in a series of earmarked federal health transfers to the provinces and territories. From the beginning, federal health transfers have been the subject of considerable debate due to differing perceptions concerning the appropriate level of health transfers and the degree of conditionality (or lack thereof) that accompanies such transfers (Lazar & St-Hilaire, 2004; Marchildon, 2004; McIntosh, 2004). Initially, federal health transfers were introduced as a 50:50 shared cost transfer to support provincial universal hospital insurance programmes beginning in 1958 and to support provincial and territorial universal medical insurance programmes a decade later. These transfers were eventually perceived by some as too restrictive in terms of their exclusive emphasis on hospital and physician expenditures, and by the federal government as overly risky from a fiscal perspective given the rapid growth in provincial and territorial medicare spending.

By 1977, the federal and provincial governments negotiated the replacement of the cost-sharing transfer with a less conditional block transfer – EPF – that merged the health transfer with another transfer fund for higher education. EPF gave the provinces greater flexibility. No longer required to spend federal money on hospitals and medical care, provincial governments could apply transfer funds to any category of health expenditure including the nonmedical determinants of health. In return, the federal government was able to cap the growth in its health transfers to the growth in the national economy rather than matching the growth in provincial health spending (Coyte & Landon, 1990; Ostry, 2006). However, there were other consequences, including the fact that the portion converted into a permanent tax point transfer could not be taken away in the event of provincial non-compliance with the conditionality in the Hospital Insurance and Diagnostic Services Act or the Medical Care Act.

While the use of user fees in medicare in some provinces predated 1977, their uses seemed to accelerate after the introduction of EPF. As a consequence, in 1979, the federal minister of health ordered an external review by Justice Emmett Hall as a "check-up on medicare" after his commission's landmark report of 1964. Concluding that extra billing and user fees were undermining the principle of universality of access, Hall recommended that the federal government take legislative action (Hall, 1980). A subsequent parliamentary committee agreed with Hall and suggested that federal transfers be withheld, on a graduated basis, where a provincial plan impeded reasonable access by permitting extra billing or user fees, and this proposal was incorporated into the Canada Health Act in 1984.

In 1995, the federal government replaced EPF with the Canada Health and Social Transfer (CHST). The new transfer folded in yet another transfer fund (for social assistance) with health and higher education but the cash portion of the transfer was reduced and the provision for automatic annual increases was eliminated. These actions triggered considerable intergovernmental acrimony as well as concerns about the impact of the changes on the national dimensions of the health system (Romanow, 2002). In response to these and other concerns, the federal government replaced this omnibus CHST with the Canada Health Transfer in 2004 and reintroduced the feature of the annual increase – now set at 6% per annum for 10 years. Estimated at C$27 billion in the fiscal year 2011–2012, the Canada Health Transfer amounts to slightly more than 20% of estimated provincial spending on health in 2011 (CIHI, 2011e).

3.3.4 Purchaser–provider relations and payments to providers

In addition to administering, funding and coordinating services provided by other organizations, most RHAs also deliver health services directly. This mix of hierarchical integration and contractual coordination means that RHAs act as both purchasers and providers, although the emphasis is more on integration than competitive contracting (as it is in the United Kingdom). The one major exception to this particular RHA model is Ontario where the fourteen RHAs, known as LHINs, do not directly provide any services. Although it might be argued that that the organizational design of regionalization in Canada creates a purchaser–provider split, there is little evidence that it was formally structured in a way to promote an internal market similar to the National Health Service reforms in the United Kingdom.

Most hospitals are funded through global budgets, either directly (by ministries of health), or indirectly through budget allocations to RHAs. In recent years, some jurisdictions in Canada have begun to experiment with alternative forms of funding mechanisms for hospital care. These include activity-based funding, with British Columbia being the first province to adopt an activity-based funding approach for hospitals on a large scale (Sutherland et al., 2011). To date, there has not been a comprehensive evaluation comparing these hospital-funding mechanisms (Sutherland, 2011a).

All provincial ministries of health continue to control physician budgets and manage prescription drug plans centrally, both of which fall outside the authority of RHAs. Long-term care facilities and organizations either have a contractual relationship with RHAs or are operated directly by RHA staff. The same applies to ambulance and palliative care organizations. In the case of the contractual arrangements, RHAs negotiate the terms of contract including the amount and terms of payment.

The major change initiated by regionalization is the shift from institution-specific and service-specific funding to one based on comprehensive funding to RHAs responsible for multiple health sectors and with the latitude to allocate funds to each sector based on the needs of a defined population (McKillop, 2004). Whether this has actually improved overall results in terms of the quality of care, efficiency or overall cost requires further study. More research is also needed concerning the precise payment methods used by RHAs and their impact on health system outcomes.

3.4 Out-of-pocket payments

Since universal medicare in Canada precludes extra billing or user fees, OOP payments are only relevant to the mixed and private health sectors. Informal payments are almost non-existent in Canada: they have not been documented in any provincial or territorial health system.

OOP payments make up more than 50% of expenditure on privately financed health services and products. In particular, OOP payments form the chief source of funding for vision care, over-the-counter pharmaceuticals and CAM.

3.5 Private health insurance

PHI is relegated to non-medicare sectors such as dental care, prescription drugs, long-term care and support, as well as a few non-medically necessary physician and hospital services. As a share of private health spending, PHI has grown relative to OOP expenditure since the late 1980s. In 2008, PHI spending per capita was C$624, and PHI was more important than OOP payments in funding prescription drugs and dental care. Of the C$20.9 billion expended through PHI in 2008, $8.5 billion was spent on prescription drugs, $6.0 billion on dental care and $1.2 billion on hospital accommodation – mainly on private rooms (CIHI, 2010b).

The majority of PHI comes in the form of employment-based group policies that are benefit plans sponsored by employers, unions, professional associations and similar organizations (Hurley & Guindon, 2008). Since this type of insurance "comes with the job", it is not "voluntary". Canadians receiving or purchasing PHI are exempt from taxation on these benefits or premiums by the federal government and all provincial governments except Quebec.

Almost all PHI in Canada would be classified as complementary to medicare (Hurley & Guindon, 2008). PHI that attempts to provide a private alternative to medicare (substitutive PHI) or faster access to medicare services (supplementary PHI) is prohibited or discouraged by a complex array of provincial laws and regulations. Six provinces – British Columbia, Alberta, Manitoba, Ontario, Quebec and Prince Edward Island – and three territories prohibit the purchase of PHI for medicare services. In the remaining four provinces, the purchase of PHI for such services is discouraged through various means, in particular by not allowing physicians to work in both public and private systems at the same time (Flood & Archibald, 2001; Marchildon, 2005).

Until recently, PHI has received relatively limited policy attention because it has been restricted to complementary insurance – covering those services not included in medicare (Hurley & Guindon, 2008). In the wake of a 2005 ruling by the Supreme Court of Canada that Quebec's law prohibiting supplementary insurance for medicare services violated Quebec's Charter of Rights in the presence of excessive waiting times for non-emergency surgery, there have been repeated calls by market advocates for PHI for medicare (Flood, Roach & Sossin, 2005; Flood, 2007).

3.6 Social insurance

Of the remaining sources of finance, the single most significant is social insurance funding from provincial workers' compensation schemes. Health benefits for work-related injuries and sickness under provincial workers' compensation plans pre-date the introduction of medicare, with the first such scheme introduced by British Columbia in 1917. Administered by provincial WCBs, these benefits are paid for by compulsory employer contributions that are set by provincial law. WCB payments for health services were estimated to be C$1.4 billion, roughly 1.5% of public health expenditures (Marchildon, 2008). Much of this is paid directly to provincial health authorities and individual health facilities and providers.

Health services provided through provincial and territorial WCBs are specifically excluded from the definition of insured health services under the Canada Health Act because they are funded under the authority of laws and administrative processes that pre-date provincial medicare plans. As a consequence, WCB clients sometimes obtain – and are often perceived to be able to obtain – medicare services in advance of other Canadians, facilitated in part by WCB fees and payments that exceed the medicare tariff. For this reason, various commissions and commentators have argued that this public form of queue jumping must eventually be redressed (Romanow, 2002; Hurley et al., 2008).

In 1997, the Government of Quebec established a social insurance drug plan funded through the compulsory payment of premiums by employers. The new law mandated employers to provide PHI to cover prescription drugs, while the provincial tax law was changed to make employee health benefits a taxable benefit, thereby eliminating the tax expenditure subsidy. At the same time, individuals without access to employment-based private drug insurance (e.g. low-wage workers, retired persons and social assistance recipients) receive basic prescription drug coverage from the provincial government (Pomey et al., 2007).

3.7 Other financing

Voluntary and charitable donations provide other sources of finance for health research as well as supportive health services for patients and their families. Numerous nongovernmental organizations – from hospitals to disease-based foundations – regularly collect donations from the public. These funds are then used to purchase capital or equipment, to provide services and to direct health research. Volunteers also donate their time and skills to public and nongovernmental health service organizations and causes. According to one decade-old estimate, the voluntary sector raises C$300 million a year for health research (Health Charities Council of Canada, 2001).

3.8 Payment mechanisms

3.9.1 Paying for health services

To the extent that hospitals are integrated in RHAs in Canada, there is no purchaser–provider split. In the case of those hospitals that contract with RHAs – for example, all hospitals in Ontario and Catholic hospitals in Western Canada – most payments are generally made on the basis of the previous year's allocation adjusted for inflation and budget growth. However, some RHAs have introduced or experimented with other modes of funding, including activity-based, patient-centred and incentive-based funding models (McKillop, 2004; Sutherland, 2011a). There has been limited study of payment systems for health care organizations in Canada.

3.9.2 Paying health workers

Most non-physician health care personnel are paid a salary to work within hierarchically directed health organizations. Within this group, regulated nurses are the most numerous. Most nurse remuneration and conditions of work are negotiated through collective bargaining by nurses' unions and province-wide employer organizations, often with provincial governments setting broad fiscal parameters. Nurse dissatisfaction with working conditions and stagnant remuneration during the provincial health reforms led to labour strife and rising sick leave by the latter part of the 1990s. Since that time, staffing levels have climbed and nurse remuneration has improved considerably as governments and health organizations have attempted to recruit nurses in a tight labour market (CIHI, 2011a).

The majority of physicians continue to be remunerated on the basis of fee for service (FFS) although alternative payment methods including capitation, blended (salary and fee) payments are also applied – most commonly salary and fee or capitation and fee. In recent years, incentive-based bonuses have become more common. While many health policy analysts have been critical of the incentives created by FFS – including the incentive for overprovision of medical services – the system remains popular among many physicians and the organizations that represent them (Grignon, Paris & Polton, 2004).

Since family physicians continue to provide the majority of primary care services in Canada, primary care reform has involved some shifts in payment systems. Provincial ministries of health have considered the advantages and disadvantages of fee for service, capitation and mixed payment systems. In addition, some ministries have also begun to implement pay for performance incentives, group-based profit sharing and fundholding systems (Léger, 2011). However, these "alternative payment systems", so-called in Canada because they pose an alternative to fee-for-service systems, should not be seen as synonymous with primary care reform (Hutchison et al., 2011). In a number of cases, alternative payment is being used to pursue objectives that have little to do with altering existing forms of primary care. In some provinces for example, alternative payments are concentrated in specialties such as cancer care and psychiatry, while in other provinces, alternative payments contracts are provided for after-hours coverage of patients in primary care settings (Glazier et al., 2009; CIHI, 2010c).

4. Physical and human resources

The non-financial inputs into the Canadian health system include buildings, equipment, information technology and the health workforce. The ability of any health system to provide timely access to quality health services depends not only on the sufficiency of physical and human resources but also on finding the appropriate balance among them (Romanow, 2002). Both the sufficiency and the balance of resources need to be adjusted continually by F/P/T governments in response to the constantly evolving technology, health care practices and health needs of Canadians.

From the mid-1970s until 2000, capital investment in hospitals declined. Small hospitals were closed in many parts of Canada and acute care services were consolidated. Despite recent reinvestments by provincial and territorial governments in hospital stock, in particular in medical equipment, imaging technologies and ICT, the number of acute care beds per capita has continued to fall, in part a result of the increase in day surgeries and discharges. While most of Canada's supply of advanced diagnostic technologies is roughly comparable to levels in other OECD countries, it scores poorly in terms of its effective use of ICT relative to other high-income countries.

After a lengthy period in the 1990s when the supply of physicians and nurses, as well as other public health care workers, contracted because of government cutbacks, the health workforce has grown since 2000. The number of private sector health professionals has seen even more substantial growth during this period. Medical and nursing faculties have expanded in order to produce more graduates. At the same time, there has been an increase in the immigration of foreign-educated doctors and nurses and lower emigration to other countries such as the United States.

4.1 Physical resources

4.1.1 Capital stock and investments

From the late 1940s until the 1960s, Canada experienced rapid growth in the number and size of hospitals through the growth in demand for inpatient care. This growth was fuelled by national hospital construction grants provided to the provinces by the federal government and by the introduction of public hospital insurance in Saskatchewan, Alberta and British Columbia by the end of the 1940s, and the remaining provinces by the end of the 1950s. This construction boom would produce an overhang of outdated hospital facilities that provincial ministries of health would have to address in subsequent decades through consolidation and closure on the one hand, and the need for additional capital investment on the other (Ostry, 2006).

By the mid-1970s, the investment in hospitals had slowed, and by the 1980s and 1990s, provincial governments were encouraging hospital consolidation with a concomitant reduction in the number of small and inefficient hospitals (Mackenzie, 2004; Ostry, 2006). As provincial governments, RHAs and hospital boards closed, consolidated and converted existing establishments in an effort to reduce operating costs and increase organizational efficiencies, there was a 20% drop in the total number of hospitals offering inpatient care from the mid-1980s until the mid-1990s (Tully & Saint-Pierre, 1997).

4.1.2 Infrastructure

The number of acute care beds per capita has fallen continuously during the past two decades. In this respect, the trend in Canada is similar to the trend observed in Australia, France, Sweden, the United Kingdom and the United States (Fig. 4.1). With the exception of two territories, all jurisdictions in Canada have experienced a very similar rate of decline in hospitalization since the mid-1990s (Table 4.1). At the same time, the average length of stay (ALOS) in Canadian hospitals has increased since at least the mid-1990s (CIHI, 2010a). As seen in Table 4.2, Canada now has a higher ALOS in hospitals, a higher occupancy rate and a lower turnover rate than the other countries.

Fig. 4.1

Acute care beds per 1 000 population in Canada and selected countries, 1990–2009

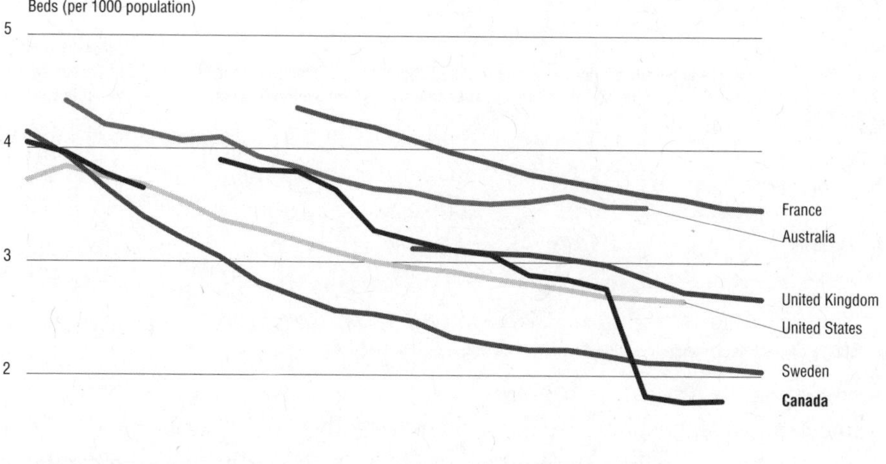

Source: OECD (2011a).
Notes: The sharp decline in 2005–2006 in Canada is due to adoption of a more consistent definition of acute care beds. From 1995 to 2005, some provinces reported rated capacity while others reported only beds staffed and in operation; from 2006, only acute care beds staffed and in operation outside of Quebec, and beds for short-term physical care in Quebec, were included (OECD, 2011b).

Table 4.1

Acute inpatient hospitalization rates (per 100 000 population) in Canada, age-standardized, 1995–1996 and 2009–2010

Province or territory	1995–1996	2009–2010	14-year change (%)
British Columbia	10 817	7 468	-31.0
Alberta	11 507	8 442	-26.6
Saskatchewan	14 764	10 953	-25.8
Manitoba	11 743	9 000	-23.4
Ontario	10 466	7 046	-32.7
Quebec	10 696	7 473	-30.1
New Brunswick	15 268	9 906	-35.1
Nova Scotia	12 033	7 762	-35.5
Prince Edward Island	14 697	10 333	-29.7
Newfoundland and Labrador	13 347	9 285	-30.4
Yukon	11 758	11 669	-0.8
Northwest Territories	20 434	14 369	-29.7
Nunavut	9 914	16 506	66.5
Canada	**11 131**	**7 706**	**-30.8**

Source: CIHI (2011e).

Table 4.2
Operating indicators for hospital-based acute care in Canada and selected countries, 2008

	Average length of stay (in days)	Number of bed days (per capita)	Occupancy rate (% of available beds)	Turnover rate (cases per available bed)
Australia	5.9	1.0	73.2	45.6
Canada	7.7	0.8	93.0	36.6
France	5.2	1.0	74.2	51.8
Sweden	4.5	–	–	–
United Kingdom	6.9	0.8	84.8	48.9
United States	5.5	0.6	66.4	44.2

Source: OECD (2011a).
Note: OECD data for bed days, occupancy rate and turnover rate for Sweden not available.

Since almost all hospital care is considered a fully insured service under the Canada Health Act, public funding is critical to decisions concerning capital expansion and improvement. Public budgeting rules require that governments and their delegates (including RHAs) carry capital expenditures as current liabilities. As a consequence, there has been an incentive to reduce capital expenditures more than operating expenditures during periods of budgetary restraint. In addition, governments sometimes prefer not to carry the burden of financing infrastructure "up front".

While some governments and RHAs have explored private finance initiatives (PFI) – known as public–private-partnerships or "P3s" in Canada – it has been more common to contract out care to private companies or professional corporations. Almost all medical laboratories and diagnostic clinics are owned by private corporations (Sutherland, 2011b).

4.1.3 Medical equipment

Canada has a decentralized process of purchasing most medical aids and devices, consistent with a decentralized delivery system. Although provincial ministries of health are ultimately responsible for ensuring the availability and quality of medical equipment, devices and aids as part of first-dollar coverage for hospital and medical services, arm's length health organizations and providers actually purchase most medical aids and devices. In addition, most physicians maintain private offices and make independent decisions concerning the purchase of a broad range of medical equipment, devices and aids to support their respective general (family) and specialist practices.

In both regionalized and non-regionalized provinces, individual clinicians, particularly specialist physicians, play a major role in the decisions of RHAs and hospitals to purchase medical equipment, including the selection of a particular vendor. At the same time, provincial health ministries can play a key role in determining the timing and procurement of extremely expensive medical equipment, especially magnetic resonance imaging (MRI) units and computed tomography (CT) scanners. From the early to mid-1990s, provincial governments severely constrained their spending on advanced diagnostics. These actions created a bottleneck, lengthening waiting times for certain conditions and treatments (Romanow, 2002). Since that time, there has been a substantial investment in advanced diagnostics by provincial health ministries and delegated RHAs. As can be seen in Table 4.3, Canada now has a supply of CT, MRI and positron emission tomography (CIHI, 2012a) scanners roughly comparable to the supply in Australia (except for CT scanners), France and the United Kingdom.

Table 4.3

Number of selected diagnostic imaging technologies, per million population, in Canada and selected countries, 2010

	CT	MRI	PET
Australia	42.5	5.8	1.4
Canada	14.4	8.4	1.2
France	11.8	7.0	0.9
United Kingdom	8.3	6.0	0.5
United States	34.3	25.9	3.1

Source: OECD (2011a).
Notes: Data for Sweden were not available; CT: Computed tomography; MRI: Magnetic resonance imaging; PET: Positron emission tomography.

Although Canada is still well below the supply of similar technologies in the United States, the simple counts of advanced technologies do not take into consideration the intensity of use, and there is evidence that advanced diagnostic technologies in Canada, particularly those that are hospital based, are more intensely used than the same imaging technologies in the United States. In fact, based on 2007 data, Canada ranked among the European countries with the highest utilization efficiency of MRI scanners, with the number of examinations per MRI in unit second only to Belgium, and higher than France, Sweden and the United Kingdom (CIHI, 2008b).

In addition, there is the question of whether some of these technologies are overused in the United States to the point that the harm caused by radiation outweighs the clinical benefit for a significant percentage of individual patients (Baker, Atlas & Afendulis, 2008; Hillman & Goldsmith, 2010). There may also be overuse in Canada driven by some primary care physicians who, as the decision-makers and gatekeepers for further care, may be referring their patients to more advanced diagnostic tests than necessary (HCC, 2010b).

Table 4.4 compares the provinces in terms of the number of selected imaging technologies per million population. There are important variations among the provinces, mostly associated with those that have smaller populations (e.g. Prince Edward Island) and, therefore, lack the economies of scale to justify investment in some high-cost technologies.

Table 4.4
Number of selected imaging technologies per million population by province, 2011

	Nuclear medicine cameras	CT scanners	MRI scanners	Angiography suites (2007 only)	Catheterization laboratories (2007 only)
British Columbia	11.8	15.2	9.3	4.8	2.8
Alberta	17.6	13.2	9.9	4.4	3.2
Saskatchewan	12.6	14.5	4.8	5.1	4.0
Manitoba	11.6	16.6	6.6	4.2	4.2
Ontario	22.2	13.6	7.7	5.8	3.9
Quebec	15.6	16.7	10.8	5.5	3.4
New Brunswick	22.6	24.0	8.0	12.0	4.0
Nova Scotia	18.4	17.4	9.8	5.4	5.4
Prince Edward Island	7.1	14.3	7.1	–	–
Newfoundland and Labrador	15.5	25.3	5.8	5.9	3.9

Source: CIHI (2012a).
Note: 2007 data only for angiography suites and catheterization laboratories (most recent available).

4.1.4 Information technology

As in all countries, access to the Internet – at home, work and school – has increased dramatically in recent years. Moreover, there is considerable evidence from a number of sources that Canadians use the Internet on a regular basis to access both medical and health information (Middleton, Veenhof & Leith, 2010).

However, in terms of ICT infrastructure, intensity of access and skill levels, it appears that Canada is not faring as well as other high-income countries, including its health system comparators. Based on a composite index of 11 indicators measuring ICT access, use and skills, the ICT Development Index, or IDI as it is known, was developed by the United Nations' International Telecommunication Union. In 2010, Canada was ranked in 26th position on this index, considerably lower than Australia, France, Sweden, the United Kingdom and the United States. Moreover, it is the only country in this group to experience a decline in its IDI ranking between 2008 and 2010 (see Table 4.5). It is also worth noting that there was a larger rural–urban gap in terms of individual use of the Internet in Canada than in Australia or the United States (ITU, 2011).

Table 4.5

ICT Development Index (IDI) based on 11 indicators, rank and level, in Canada and selected countries, 2008 and 2010

	IDI level in 2008	IDI rank in 2008	IDI level in 2010	IDI rank in 2010
Australia	6.78	14	7.36	14
Canada	6.42	20	6.69	26
France	6.55	18	7.09	18
Sweden	7.53	2	8.23	2
United Kingdom	7.03	10	7.60	10
United States	6.55	17	7.09	17

Source: ITU (2011).

Canada's performance in the use of ICT for health delivery is also poor relative to a number of other developed countries. In a 2009 survey of high-income countries that included Australia, France, Sweden, the United Kingdom and the United States, the Commonwealth Fund found that Canadian family doctors scored the lowest in terms of using EHRs and had the lowest electronic information functionality based on 14 categories among family doctors in the 11-country comparison (Schoen, et al., 2009). These results, some of which are summarized in Table 4.6, are consistent with a different survey of primary care physicians that included Germany, New Zealand, the Netherlands, Canada, Australia, the United Kingdom and the United States. In that study, Canadian physicians were again at the bottom of the league, with only 16% using some form of EHRs (Jha et al., 2008). However, based on the 2010 results of a national physician survey showing that 34% of Canadian physicians use a combination of paper and electronic records (and 16% use only electronic records), it appears that this take-up rate is improving (CIHI, 2011f).

Table 4.6
Use of health IT by primary care physicians (% of physicians), 2009

	Electronic patient medical records	Routine electronic access to patient test results	Routine electronic prescribing of medication	Routine electronic alerts prompting problem with drug dose or interaction	Routine electronic ordering of laboratory tests	Routine electronic entry of clinical notes	Computerized capacity to generate list of patients by diagnosis	Computerized capacity to generate list of patients overdue for tests or preventative care	Computerized capacity to generate lists of all medications taken by patient
Australia	95	93	93	92	86	92	93	95	94
Canada	37	41	27	20	18	30	37	22	25
France	68	36	57	43	40	60	20	19	24
Sweden	94	91	93	58	81	89	74	41	49
UK	96	89	89	93	35	97	90	89	86
US	46	59	40	37	38	42	42	29	30

Source: Schoen et al. (2009).

Although data are very limited on the use of health IT in hospital settings, it does appear that the adoption and use of ICT in Canadian hospitals is also limited. In a domestic survey of hospitals in five provinces and two territories, Urowitz et al. (2008) found that a bare majority had some sort of EHRs while only a small minority (2.4%) had records with an electronic content between 91% and 100%.

The WHO's more recent set of profiles on e-health in 114 participating countries paints a somewhat more positive picture of the state of health information in Canada, although the WHO (2011a) did not attempt a numeric assessment or comparison of country performance. Although a report by the Auditor General of Canada (2009) provides a limited but largely positive assessment of the accountability performance of Canada Health Infoway, there remains an obvious need for a rigorous analysis of the extent and effectiveness of health IT in Canada.

4.2 Human resources

4.2.1 Health workforce trends

During the past decade, P/T government decision-makers throughout Canada have expressed concerns about health human resource shortages, in particular doctors and nurses. In response, these governments implemented policies to increase educational enrolments as well as recruit professionals from outside their respective jurisdictions and from other countries. This shift contrasts with the period in the early to mid-1990s when governments were concerned about surpluses and actively worked with the professions and postsecondary institutions to curtail the supply of both physicians and nurses as well as reduce the number of new entrants into these professions (Tuohy, 2002; Chan, 2002a; Evans & McGrail, 2008).

At a minimum, these efforts have produced higher health sector remuneration and inflation (CIHI, 2011b). They are also increasing the per capita supply of nurses and doctors. However, it is important to note that while doctor density surpassed 1990 levels by 2009, nurse density continued to decline substantially after 2000, and had not recovered to 1990 levels even by 2009 (see Table 4.7).

Table 4.7

Practising health professionals in Canada per 1 000 population, selected years, 1990–2009

	1990	1995	2000	2005	2009
Nurses	11.10	10.89	10.13	8.71	9.39
Primary care doctors	1.06	1.03	1.00	1.04	1.12
Medical group of specialists	0.41	0.43	0.45	0.47	0.53
Surgical group of specialists	0.34	0.33	0.34	0.33	0.36
Psychiatrists	0.13	0.14	0.14	0.15	0.15
Dentists	0.52	0.53	0.56	0.58	0.59
Pharmacists	0.68	0.70	0.77	0.79	0.88
Physiotherapists	–	–	–	0.50	0.52

Source: OECD (2011a).

Other health professions were not affected by the budgetary constraints of F/P/T governments in the early to mid-1990s. Since dental care is largely private in Canada, dentists were not affected by public-sector expenditure cutting in the 1990s. While prescription drugs are a mixed sector subject to both public and private coverage and, therefore, insulated to a limited degree by public budget cutting, the more salient factor affecting the number of pharmacists has been the rapid increase in drug utilization during the past two decades.

Due to geography, population dispersion and differences in health systems and policies, there are significant variations in the density of the health professions among provinces and territories. As illustrated in Table 4.8, the RN density in the Northwest Territories and Nunavut is considerably higher than the Canadian average, while the physician density is considerably lower. This is a product of dispersed Arctic communities that rely heavily on nurse-based primary care provided in publicly administered health centres rather than on family physicians. With the exception of a large presence in the three northern territories, the populations of which suffer most from dental disease, the dental professions tend to concentrate in the four most urbanized provinces in Canada – Ontario, Quebec, British Columbia and Alberta.

Table 4.8

Health workforce density by province and territory, rate per 100 000 population, 2009

Province/territory	Nurses		Physicians		Dental professionals			Others			
	RNs	LPNs	Primary	Specialists	Dentists	Dental hygienists	Pharmacists	Optometrists	Physiotherapists	Occupational therapists	Psychologists
British Columbia	688	169	119	96	67	63	88	11	59	36	25
Alberta	792	180	113	91	54	62	100	13	54	41	67
Saskatchewan	878	253	94	72	37	40	115	12	51	25	46
Manitoba	907	216	95	88	51	50	100	9	56	41	17
Ontario	718	219	90	97	63	81	79	13	49	32	25
Quebec	839	244	110	112	54	61	95	17	48	52	95
New Brunswick	1 048	364	109	85	39	48	92	15	60	40	41
Nova Scotia	949	357	117	115	56	58	117	11	60	40	49
Prince Edward Island	996	471	89	76	50	51	114	13	38	31	20
Newfoundland and Labrador	1 140	494	118	102	35	23	116	10	38	30	39
Yukon	1 080	188	190	30	142	75	85	15	103	[26]	–
Northwest Territories	[1 348]	217	69	30	113	51	46	0	–	[26]	180
Nunavut	[1 348]	–	31	–	156	6	92	25	–	[26]	60
Canada	**785**	**227**	**103**	**99**	**58**	**67**	**90**	**14**	**51**	**39**	**47**

Source: CIHI (2011d).
Notes: numbers in square parentheses indicate areas where a single estimate was made for RNs (NWT + NU) and occupational therapists (YK + NWT + NU) for a larger northern region; LPNs: Licensed registered practical nurse .

During the 1990s, physician supply grew at an annual average of 1.1% – a rate that would more than double from 2004 to 2009 due in part to the rapid expansion of places in Canadian medical schools and the influx of international medical graduates (Watanabe, Comeau & Buske, 2008; CIHI, 2011b). As a consequence, the number of physicians per capita has begun to rise in recent years, a trend already apparent in Australia, France, Sweden, the United Kingdom and the United States well before the increase in Canada (Fig. 4.2).

Fig. 4.2

Number of physicians per 1 000 population in Canada and selected countries, 1990–2010

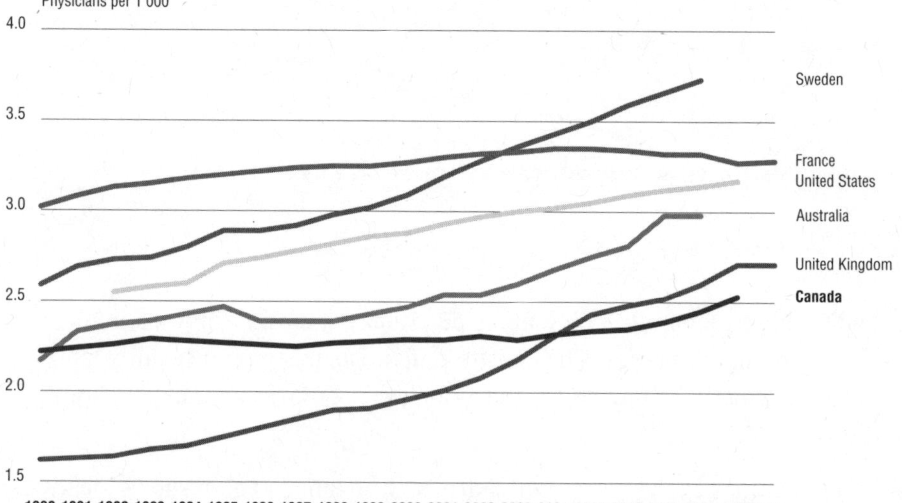

Source: OECD (2011a).
Note: In order to create a time series, it was necessary to use data for Australia, Sweden and the United States based on practising physicians, while data for Canada, France and the United Kingdom are based on physicians licensed to practice.

When comparing Canada with its five OECD comparators in terms of the number of nurses per 1000 population, it appears that only Australia witnessed a comparable decline in the density of nurses in the 1990s. By 2005, the trend had reversed in Canada, and the ratio of nurses to population has increased since that time (Fig. 4.3).

Fig. 4.3
Number of nurses per 1 000 population in Canada and selected countries, 1990–2010

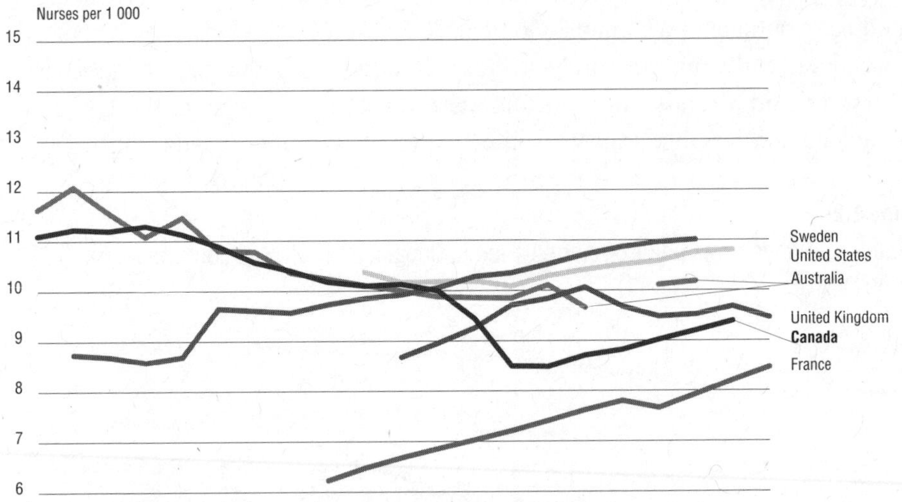

Source: OECD (2011a).
Note: Data for Australia, Canada and the United Kingdom are limited to non-administrative practising nurses, while data for France, Sweden and the United States include nurses working in administration, management or research.

The trend in the number of dentists per 1000 population shows a marked contrast with that of nurses. The density of dentists has grown steadily since 1990, a trend shared by only Australia among the countries in the comparator group (Fig. 4.4).

When it comes to the density of pharmacists, Canada again shows steady growth in the last two decades. As can be seen in Fig. 4.5, this density level is similar to the comparator countries. The one exception is France, where the population has historically been among the largest consumers of prescription drugs in the world (Chevreul et al., 2010).

Fig. 4.4

Number of dentists per 1 000 population in Canada and selected countries, 1990–2010

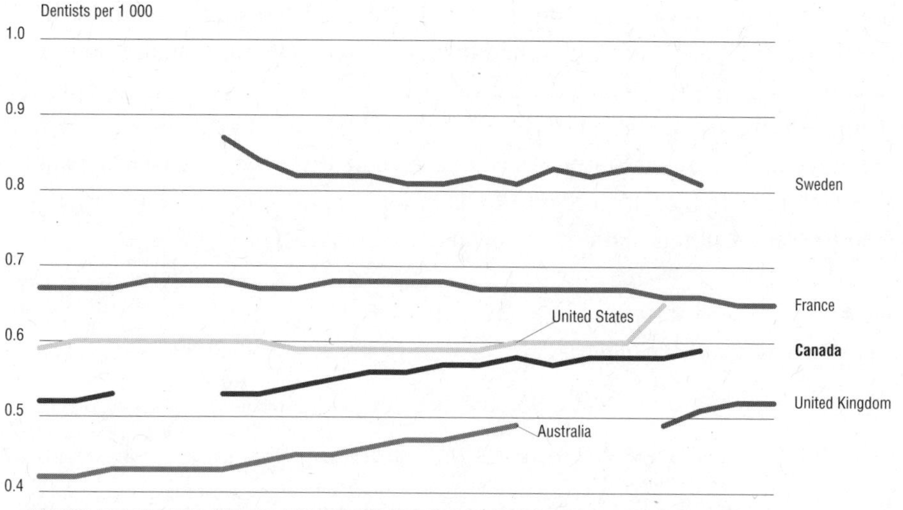

Source: OECD (2011a).
Note: Data for Australia, Canada, France and United States are limited to practising dentists, while data for Sweden and the United Kingdom include dentists working in administration and management positions.

Fig. 4.5

Number of pharmacists per 1 000 population in Canada and selected countries, 1990–2010

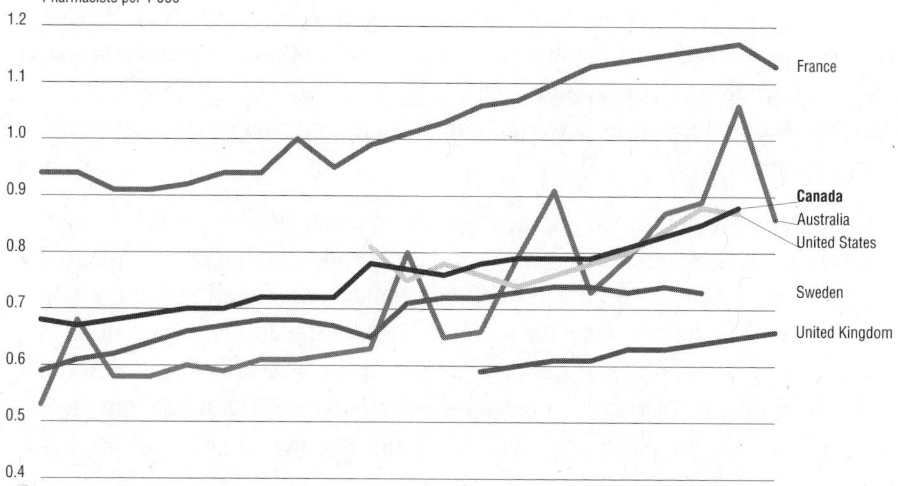

Source: OECD (2011a).
Note: Data for Australia, Sweden and the United Kingdom are limited to practising pharmacists, while data for Canada, France and the United States include pharmacists working in administration and research.

4.2.2 Professional mobility of health workers

Physicians are highly mobile in Canada and the competition for physicians among and within provincial and territorial health systems has been intense since the late 1990s. This has resulted in significant inter-provincial mobility. Two-thirds of physicians who leave a province or territory move to another part of Canada rather than abroad (CIHI, 2010d). When doctors do move abroad, most move to the United States. As can be seen in Table 4.9, there has been a steady net migration of doctors into Canada for the past three decades largely due to the influx of international medical graduates (IMGs).

Table 4.9
Net international migration of physicians, Canada, by decade, 1980–2009

Decade	Moved abroad	Returned from abroad	New IMGs	Net migration	Average annual impact on stock of physicians (%)
1980–1989	3 244	1 806	5 216	3 778	0.9
1990–1999	5 541	2 091	4 755	1 305	0.2
2000–2009	2 859	2 000	7 181	6 322	1.0

Source: CIHI (2010d).

Although the overall impact of migration appears to have had a marginal impact on the overall domestic supply of physicians, Table 4.9 obscures the extent to which some provinces are highly reliant on IMGs: for example, in the past decade, almost 50% of new physicians in Saskatchewan are foreign educated, the majority from developing countries, especially South Africa. Indeed, some ministries of health in association with the provincial medical bodies have established programmes to facilitate and speed up the licensure of IMGs, many of whom, at least initially, migrate to underserviced areas in the country (Dumont et al., 2008).

Nurses are also mobile and the shortage of nurses has intensified competition among the provinces, territories, RHAs and independent hospitals over the past decade. As a consequence, salaries and wages have risen well above the rate of salaries outside the health sector (CIHI, 2011b). In the 2000s, approximately 7–8% of the nurse workforce was originally educated outside Canada. Some jurisdictions and health organizations have actively recruited nurses from other countries, such as the Philippines (CIHI, 2010d; Runnels, Labonte & Packer, 2011).

The hiring of international medical and nursing graduates has raised concerns about the impact of this practice on developing countries. Estimates of the public cost of educating a doctor in nine sub-Sahara African countries, for example, range from a low of $21 000 in Uganda to a high of US $58 700 in South Africa (Mills et al., 2011). These are countries with great health needs and limited resources to educate and train doctors, which has led to the charge that such foreign recruitment may be unethical (McIntosh, Torgerson & Klassen, 2007; Runnels, Labonte & Packer, 2011).

4.2.3 Education and training of health workers

In terms of educating and training health providers, provincial ministries of health work in tandem with provider organizations to set or alter the number of "seats" or entry positions in professional programmes in postsecondary institutions. Since education is exclusively within the jurisdiction of the provinces and almost all education in Canada is financed publicly, provincial governments determine the funding for the postsecondary education of the health professions that is delivered by universities, colleges and technical institutions (Tzountzouris & Gilbert, 2009). Table 4.10 sets out the educational and training requirements for 22 health occupations.

There are 17 medical programmes offering a medical doctorate (MD) in Canadian universities. The programmes vary in length from three years (McMaster University and University of Calgary) to the more typical four-year programme including the clinical practicum (CIHI, 2011a). After graduating, medical students enter a residency programme in family practice or some specialization and complete their training – a minimum two-year residency programme in the case of family practice and four or more years in other specialties in medical, surgical and laboratory medicine. As in most countries, the number of physician specialties has grown over time. As of 2011, there were 28 specialties, 36 subspecialties and two special programmes for a total of 66 individual study and training programmes. A small number of physician assistants (250 as of 2011) work in Manitoba and Ontario, the two provinces that also offer university-based programmes for these physician extenders.

Table 4.10

Educational and training requirements of 22 health occupations, 2009

Occupation	Minimum education required	Internship or clinical practicum required	National examination (in addition to any P/T requirements)
Audiologist	Master's	Yes	Yes
Chiropractor	Professional doctorate	Yes	Yes
Dental hygienist	Diploma	Yes	Yes
Dentist	Professional doctorate	Yes	Yes
Dietician	Bachelor's	Yes	Yes
Environmental public health professional	Bachelor's	Yes	Yes
Health information management professional	Diploma or Bachelor's	Yes	Yes
Licensed practical nurse	Diploma	Yes	Yes
Medical laboratory technologist	Diploma	Yes	Yes
Medical radiation technologist	Diploma	Yes	Yes
Midwife	Bachelor's	Yes	Yes
Nurse practitioner	Master's or Post-Bachelor's Certificate	Yes	Yes
Occupational therapist	Master's	Yes	Yes
Optometrist	Professional doctorate	Yes	Yes
Pharmacist	Bachelor's	Yes	Yes
Physician	Medical doctorate plus residency	Yes	Yes
Physiotherapist	Master's	Yes	Yes
Psychologist	Doctorate	Yes	Yes
RN	Diploma or Bachelor's	Yes	Yes
Registered psychiatric nurse	Diploma or Bachelor's	Yes	Yes
Respiratory therapist	Diploma	Yes	Yes
Speech–language pathologist	Master's	Yes	Yes

Source: Compiled from CIHI (2011a).

While undergraduate education and the awarding of undergraduate medical degrees (the basic "medical doctorate") is the purview of the 17 medical schools in Canada, the RCPSC is responsible for overseeing the graduate education and training of physicians. As such, the RCPSC accredits 17 residency programmes, all run by the university-based medical schools. Specialists are also certified by the RCPSC, which is recognized by all province medical licensing authorities except for Quebec, where the Collège des médecins du Québec is the primary certifying body (Flegel, Hébert & MacDonald, 2008; Bates, Lovato & Buller-Taylor, 2008; CIHI, 2011a).

Educational requirements for nurses have increased dramatically over the last two decades, with a major shift from two-year diploma programmes to four-year bachelor degree programmes. Nurse practitioners are RNs whose extra training and education entitles them to an "extended class" designation. Their scope of practice – which includes prescribing certain classes of prescription drug and ordering some diagnostic tests – overlaps with that of family physicians. More importantly, given the evidence of the declining comprehensiveness of the primary care offered by physicians since the late 1980s, the range of health services offered by nurse practitioners has been of interest to primary health care reform advocates and provincial ministries of health (Chan, 2002b; College of Nurses of Ontario, 2004; CIHI, 2011c). In addition to their RN education and training, nurse practitioners must get additional training from accredited institutions that are offered in all ten provinces. The length of these programmes, including the clinical practicum, vary from one year to slightly in excess of two years (CIHI, 2011a).

To practise in Canada, a pharmacist must hold a bachelor's degree in pharmacy from an accredited programme, pass the qualifying examination administered by the Pharmacy Examining Board of Canada, and register with the appropriate P/T regulatory body. Ten universities offer programmes in Canada. All are four-year programmes, including clinical practicum, with the exception of a five-year programme at Memorial University of Newfoundland. There have been between 705 and 1075 pharmacy graduates a year from these Canadian universities between 2000 and 2009 (CIHI, 2011a).

Chiropractors in Canada must have a doctorate of chiropractic (DC) from an accredited programme, pass the Canadian Chiropractors Examining Board National Competency Examination and register with a provincial or territorial regulatory body as required. There are two accredited chiropractic programmes in Canada: a four-year programme at the Canadian Memorial Chiropractic College in Ontario, and a five-year programme at the Université du Québec à Trois-Rivières in Quebec, which together have produced between 188 and 218 graduates a year between 2000 and 2009 (CIHI, 2011a).

Dentists practising in Canada must have a doctor of dental medicine (DDM) or a doctor of dental surgery (DDS) degree from an accredited programme, pass the National Dental Examining Board of Canada Written Examination and Objective Structured Clinical Examination as well as register with the pertinent P/T regulatory body. There are ten accredited programmes, all four years in length. There is considerable competition for entry into Canada's ten dental schools, five of which are located in Quebec and Ontario. Canadians are among the world's highest spenders on dental care, in part due to the prevalence of private dental insurance – largely through employment-based benefit plans. As with physicians, a number of specializations requiring two to three years of higher education and residency have emerged over time including (but not limited to) orthodontists, periodontists, endodontists and paediatric dentists. A number of allied dental professionals support dentists and dental specialists in their work, including dental asssistants, dental hygienists and dental therapists. Provincial dental organizations are responsible for licensing and self-regulating various professional subgroups, although the Royal College of Dentists of Canada plays a role similar to the RCPSC in setting standards for postgraduate education and training.

4.2.4 Career paths

There are few formalized managerial and policy career paths for clinicians, including doctors and nurses, within the health system. This is despite the fact that, increasingly, clinicians are asked to take on managerial roles within health systems. As a consequence, career paths are being developed but in an ad hoc and varying manner by individual health care organizations.

Originally established in 1970, the Canadian College of Health Leaders – originally known as the Canadian College of Health Service Executives – provides professional support including a journal, professional programmes and services. It also offers a competency-based "Certified Health Executive" programme for its members, some of whom include existing and former clinicians.

5. Provision of services

Although it is difficult to generalize given the decentralized nature of health services administration and delivery in Canada, the typical patient pathway starts with a visit to a family physician, who then determines the course of basic treatment, if any. Family physicians act as gatekeepers: they decide whether their patients should obtain diagnostic tests, prescription drug therapies or be referred to medical specialists. However, provincial ministries of health have renewed efforts to reform primary care in the last decade. Many of these reform efforts focus on moving from the traditional physician-only practice to interprofessional primary care teams that provide a broader range of primary health care services on a 24-hour, 7-day-a-week basis. In cases where the patient does not have a regular family physician or needs help after regular clinic hours, the first point of contact may be a walk-in medical clinic or a hospital emergency department.

Illness prevention services including disease screening may be provided by a family physician, a public health office or within a dedicated screening programme. All provincial and territorial governments have public health and health promotion initiatives. They also conduct health surveillance and manage epidemic response. While PHAC develops and manages programmes supporting public health throughout Canada, most day-to-day public health activities and supporting infrastructure remains with the provincial and territorial governments.

Almost all acute care is provided in public or non-profit-making private hospitals in Canada, although some specialized ambulatory and advanced diagnostic services may be provided in private profit-making clinics. Most hospitals have an emergency department that is fed by independent emergency medical service units providing first response care to patients while being transported to emergency departments.

As for prescription drugs, every provincial and territorial government has a prescription drug plan that covers outpatient prescription drugs for designated populations (e.g. seniors and social assistance recipients), with the federal government providing drug coverage for eligible First Nations and Inuit. These public insurers depend heavily on HTA, including the CDR conducted by the CADTH, to determine which drugs should be included in their respective formularies. Despite the creation of a National Pharmaceuticals Strategy following the 10-Year Plan agreed by first ministers in 2004, there has been little progress on a pan-Canadian catastrophic drug coverage programme.

Rehabilitation and long-term care policies and services, including home and community care, palliative care and support for informal carers, vary considerably among provinces and territories. Until the 1960s, the locus of most mental health care was in large, provincially run psychiatric hospitals. Since deinstitutionalization, individuals with mental illnesses are diagnosed and treated by psychiatrists on an outpatient basis even though they may spend periods of time in the psychiatric wards of hospitals. Family physicians provide the majority of primary mental health care.

Unlike mental health care, almost all dental care is privately funded in Canada. As a consequence of access being largely based on income, outcomes are highly inequitable. CAM is also privately funded and delivered.

Due to the disparities in health outcomes for Aboriginal peoples – as well as the historical challenge of servicing some of the most remote communities in Canada – F/P/T governments have established a number of targeted programmes and services. While Aboriginal health status has improved in the postwar period, a large gap in health status continues to separate the Aboriginal population from most other Canadians.

5.1 Public health

Public health aims to improve health, prolong life and improve the quality of life through health promotion, disease prevention and other forms of health intervention. Unlike the other services covered in this chapter, the majority of public health policies and programmes target populations rather than individuals. Provincial governments have had a long history of public health interventions dating back to 1882 when Ontario's Public Health Act established a broad range of public health measures, a permanent board of health and the country's first medical officer of health.

In Canada, public health is generally identified with the following six discrete functions: population health assessment, health promotion, disease and injury control and prevention, health protection, surveillance and emergency preparedness and epidemic response. The F/P/T governments (and their delegated authorities including RHAs) perform some or all of these functions. All governments appoint a chief public or medical health officer to lead their public health efforts in their respective jurisdictions. These individuals are generally physicians with specialized education and training in public health.

By virtue of their extensive responsibilities for health and health care, provincial ministries of health all have public health branches (some even have a separate public health agency or department) with responsibility for the six discrete functions of public health. In addition, most ministries of health have launched major population health initiatives in recent years. In some provinces, RHAs have initiated their own public health promotion and illness prevention programmes in areas of greatest need for their respective populations.

The federal government also provides a broad range of public health services principally through PHAC, which coordinates, at least in part, the six public health functions described above. PHAC is responsible for disease surveillance including reporting back to the WHO and other relevant international bodies. PHAC also administers a network of disease-control laboratory services such as the National Microbiology Laboratory. Like Health Canada, PHAC is responsible for funding and administering a number of public health programmes, some of which emphasize the social determinants of health, including the Aboriginal Head Start Program, the Canada Prenatal Nutrition Program and the Healthy Living Strategy, and illness prevention programmes for AIDS and tobacco reduction.

The CPHA is a voluntary organization dedicated to improving the state of public health in Canada. In conjunction with its provincial and territorial branches or associations, CPHA advocates for greater awareness of the impact of public health interventions and encourages public health research and education.

The provinces are mainly responsible for the funding and administration of screening programmes for the early detection of cancer, and all provincial and territorial ministries of health have implemented one or more of these programmes. Although they vary considerably in approach, delivery and comprehensiveness, provincial governments do adopt screening programmes developed in other provinces once they have proven successful. For example, British Columbia was the first province to initiate a population-based breast cancer programme in 1988. Two years later, the province of Ontario began to provide population-based breast cancer screening for women aged 50 or older. Following this, the Canadian Breast Cancer Screening Initiative was launched with funding support from Health Canada, and a pan-Canadian breast screening surveillance database was established based on provincial data. Organized breast cancer screening is now the norm rather than the exception in Canada (Cancer Care Ontario, 2010; PHAC, 2011). It is estimated that screening contributed to roughly half of the reduction in breast cancer mortality in Canada between 1986 and 2005 (Wadden, 2005). Cervical cancer screening and surveillance followed a very similar trajectory in the 1990s.

In the 2000s, there has been a major effort to improve and extend screening for colorectal cancer, the second leading cause of cancer mortality in Canada. By 2004, clinical guidelines had been established for colorectal cancer testing. In 2007, based on the success of an earlier pilot project, the government of Ontario established a province-wide, population-based colorectal cancer screening programme, the same year that the Government of Manitoba set up its own organized screening pilot project. One year later, a large sample of Canadians was asked if they had received the recommended colorectal cancer testing to determine the impact of population-based as opposed to physician-based screening (Table 5.1). Although self-reported results must be treated cautiously, they did indicate substantially higher levels of screening in Ontario and Manitoba and will most likely encourage other provinces to institute population-based screening for colorectal cancer.

All provincial and territorial ministries of health also devote resources to communicable and infectious disease control. However, given the geographical reach of such diseases and the rapidity with which they spread, the federal government has begun to play a larger role in both control and surveillance. The SARS (severe acute respiratory syndrome) outbreak in 2003 and the advisory report that followed in its wake were the catalysts for a policy change, which many public health advocates considered overdue (Health Canada, 2003). One year later, PHAC was established with a mandate to monitor, prepare for and respond to disease outbreaks in addition to other public health functions.

Table 5.1
Colorectal cancer testing, self-reported (% of provincial or territorial population), 2008

Province/Territory	% of population
British Columbia	37
Alberta	37
Saskatchewan	38
Manitoba	53
Ontario	50
Quebec	28
New Brunswick	34
Nova Scotia	32
Prince Edward Island	32
Newfoundland and Labrador	34
Yukon (territory)	29
Northwest Territories	30
Nunavut	–

Source: Wilkins & Shields (2009).
Note: Residents were asked whether they had had a faecal occult blood test in the past two years or a colonoscopy or signoidoscopy in the past five years. The sample size for Nunavut was too small for a reliable result.

Immunization planning and programming is also a primary responsibility for provincial and territorial health ministries (De Wals, 2011). Immunization can be delivered in a number of ways but the two most common are through family physicians or regionally based public health offices. The National Advisory Committee on Immunizations is a pan-Canadian committee of recognized experts that works with, and reports the results of its deliberations to PHAC. Its recommendations are conveyed to the public, including health providers and health system decision-makers, in the *Canadian Immunization Guide,* which is published every five years (NACI, 2006).

5.2 Patient pathways

Due to the decentralized nature of health delivery, patient pathways vary considerably depending on the province or territory of residents. The following steps are part of a highly stylized pathway of a woman named Mary living in the more southern and urban part of the country:[1]

[1] In the far north of the provinces and in the three northern territories, the first point of contact is more likely to be an RN in a community health centre.

1. On getting ill, Mary visits her family physician where she is given a preliminary examination. Depending on the diagnosis, Mary could be given a prescription for a drug therapy, a referral for further diagnostic tests or a referral to a specialist. Mary does not pay for her physician visits or the cost of any physician-ordered, medically necessary diagnostic tests.
2. If given a prescription, Mary will go to a drug store of her choice and give the pharmacist the prescription signed by her physician. If she does not have private insurance or does not meet the requirements of her provincial drug plan, Mary may have to pay the full cost of the drug.
3. If sent for further diagnostic tests, Mary will provide blood or other bodily fluids at a private laboratory or get basic (e.g. radiography) or advanced (e.g. MRI) diagnostic tests either at a private clinic or a hospital. Since these tests are medically necessary, Mary will not be charged a fee irrespective of where she obtains the test.
4. Mary's diagnostics results will be returned to the family physician. Once the physician receives the results, she or he will call Mary back to his or her office for a further consultation and, if necessary, explain the next steps in treatment.
5. If referred to a specialist (consulting) physician, Mary will be examined and a decision made concerning specialized treatment. Her family physician will be informed of the results.
6. If the treatment involves a surgical procedure or other acute intervention, Mary will be given a date to attend the hospital or, in cases involving more routine day surgeries, a specialized surgery clinic.
7. On Mary's discharge from the hospital, her family physician receives a discharge summary from her specialist to allow for appropriate follow-up.
8. If Mary requires further home care or rehabilitation services, Mary's doctor will provide a referral. If these services are deemed medically necessary by her physician, she will not pay; otherwise, she may pay part or all of the costs, depending on the coverage offered in her province of residence.

5.3 Primary/ambulatory care

Primary care is defined as the individual's first point of contact with the health system and, at its core, involves general medical care for common conditions and injuries. It can, and should, involve some health promotion and disease prevention activities although, unlike the public health services described above, these will be provided at the individual rather than population level. Ambulatory care refers to non-acute medical services provided to an individual who is not confined to an institutional bed as an inpatient during the time the services are provided. However, in Canada, since most specialized ambulatory care tends to be provided in a hospital on a day surgery basis, this type of care is dealt with as part of inpatient care in the following section.

The traditional model of primary care in Canada has been one based on individual family physicians providing primary medical services on a fee-for-service basis. While rostering or other forms of patient enrolment or registration are not generally used, most family physicians have a relatively stable group of patients after the initial period required to build up a medical practice. And while patients are free to change their family physicians, most choose to have long-standing relationships with one physician.

In the 1970s and 1980s, provinces and territories established a number of initiatives to improve primary care, including the establishment of community-based primary care clinics in Ontario and Quebec. By the 1990s, there were a number of primary health care reforms initiated on a pilot basis. Despite this activity and earlier reforms, there was limited change by the end of the century (Hutchison, Abelson & Lavis, 2001). In the past ten years, there has been a renewed effort by provincial and territorial ministries to achieve some concrete improvements in primary health care.

In the 10-Year Plan of 2004 (see section 6.1), all provincial and territorial governments committed themselves to ensuring that at least 50% of their respective residents would have access to primary care 24 hours a day, 7 days a week, commonly referred to as 24/7 access. Some jurisdictions have set targets concerning the replacement of fee-for-service remuneration by alternative payment contracts that encourage more time spent on consultation and diagnosis. Other jurisdictions are experimenting with different models of primary care delivery although most of the reforms are more evolutionary than revolutionary (Hutchison et al., 2011).

The government of Ontario now has a number of different primary care practice models that are being assessed in terms of performance (ICES, 2012). These include the community health centres, a salaried model that services lower socioeconomic status populations; the family health groups based on a blended fee-for-service model; the family health networks and Family Health Organizations whose physicians are funded on a blended capitation model; and the family health teams which are made up of several types of professionals, the physician members being funded on a blended capitation model. The Institute of Clinical Evaluative Sciences compared all five models in terms of emergency department visits in one year (2008/9–2009/10), and found that patients/clients enrolled in the community health centres and family health groups had considerably fewer emergency department visits that those enrolled with the family health organizations, the family health teams, and the family health networks (ICES, 2012).

5.4 Inpatient care/specialized ambulatory care

In Canada, virtually all secondary, tertiary and emergency care, as well as the majority of specialized ambulatory care, is performed in hospitals. Based on the typology introduced by Healy & McKee (2002), the prevailing trend for decades has been towards the separatist model of acute care rather than a comprehensive model of hospital-based curative care. In the separatist model, the hospital specializes in acute and emergency care, leaving primary care to family physicians or community-based health care clinics and institutional care to long-term care homes and similar facilities. There are important exceptions and variations in Canada. In British Columbia, for example, a great deal of long-term care has been attached to hospitals. However, a clearly noticeable trend in Canada is for the consolidation of tertiary care in fewer, more specialized, hospitals, as well as the spinning off of some types of elective surgery and advanced diagnostics to specialized clinics.

Historically, hospitals in Canada were organized and administered on a local basis, and almost all were administered at arm's length from provincial governments (Boychuk, 1999; Deber, 2004). In the provinces and territories that have regionalized, hospitals have been integrated into a broader continuum of care either through direct RHA ownership or through contract with RHAs. Where the hospital is owned by the RHAs, the hospital boards have been disbanded and senior management are employees of the RHA. If the hospital is owned by religious or secular civil society organization – generally a non-profit-making organization with charitable status – it continues to have a board and senior management that is independent of the RHA. However, since independent hospitals derive most of their income stream from the RHAs, they generally conform to the overall objectives of the RHA and are integrated to a considerable degree into the RHA's continuum of care services.

Specialized ambulatory services are generally provided in outpatient departments of hospitals. Although there is a noticeable trend towards providing such services in specialized clinics and physician practices, this has not yet become the dominant mode of delivery in part because of the public reaction to switching from delivery by non-profit-making hospitals to delivery by profit-making clinics. Organized labour, in particular, has been hostile to this development since it may involve moving from a unionized workforce to a non-unionized workforce, and one of the largest public sector unions in Canada, the Canadian Union of Public Employees, has been vocal in its opposition to private-sector contracting out (Canadian Union of Public Employees, 2005). In addition, the Canadian Health Coalition, a civil society organization dedicated to defending universal medicare in Canada, has also lobbied against provincial privatization initiatives including hospital public-private partnerships (P3s in Canada) (Shrybman, 2007).

5.5 Emergency care

Emergency care in Canada generally refers to the care provided in an emergency department, sometimes also referred to as an emergency ward or emergency room, of a hospital, staffed for 24 hours a day by emergency physicians and emergency nurses. Emergency care also includes the emergency medical services that provide transportation (e.g. road or air ambulance) and the pre-hospital or inter-hospital patient care during transportation, including the certified first responders and emergency medical technicians who stabilize the patient before and during transportation. Physicians who practise emergency medicine are either specialist fellows of the RCPSC or specialist family physicians who are certified through the College of Family Physicians of Canada. RNs can be certified as emergency nurses through the Canadian Nurses Association.

There has been much concern about ED overcrowding and long waiting times in the past decade. In a 2004–2005 survey, 62% of ED directors perceived overcrowding to be a major or severe problem (CADTH, 2006). The evidence, although limited, supports the prevalent perception that the time from ED triage to treatment has increased significantly and the time patients spend in ED departments has also increased steadily (Bullard et al., 2009).

In Canada, a man with acute appendicitis on a Sunday morning would take the following steps:

1. The man goes directly to the ED (the vast majority of ED patients come without a GP's referral). He is taken to hospital by a household member or by an ambulance.
2. Once at the ED, he provides his provincial health card and briefly describes the problem. He is then referred to a triage nurse who estimates the urgency of the complaint after further inquiry. The waiting time for admission into an ED room for further tests and examination depends on the level of urgency.
3. The man is then examined by an emergency physician and told about the diagnosis and the recommended surgical procedure.
4. A medical team performs the required surgery or procedure.

5.6 Pharmaceutical care

Inpatient drugs are dispensed by hospitals without charge to patients as part of medicare. Outpatient pharmaceuticals, the cost of which may be covered in whole or part through public or private drug plans, are prescribed by physicians and in rare cases by other health providers who have the right to prescribe certain classes of drugs. Individuals obtain their prescription drugs at retail pharmacies. Almost all pharmacies, whether they are independent or part of a chain, sell a host of products beyond prescription and over-the-counter drugs. Pharmacies in large chain grocery stores now compete directly with traditional stand-alone pharmacies by selling prescription and over-the-counter drugs.

Provincial and territorial drug plans vary in terms of the extent and depth of coverage, and these variations are most pronounced for expensive drugs (Menon, Stafinski & Stuart, 2005; Grootendorst & Hollis, 2011; McLeod et al., 2011). Unlike all other provincial plans, the Quebec drug programme is a mandated social insurance plan in which the private sector plays a key role (Pomey et al., 2007). To add further complexity to these provincial and territorial differences, eligible First Nations and Inuit patients are covered through the federal non-insured health benefits programme. The one exception is inpatient drug therapy: since prescription drugs provided in hospitals are considered part of universal coverage, they are provided to all provincial and territorial residents, including First Nations and Inuit, free of charge, by P/T governments.

In terms of public and private insurance coverage for prescription drugs, there is an east–west gradient in Canada, with residents living in the four Western Canadian provinces as well as Ontario and Quebec having noticeably deeper coverage than residents living in the four Atlantic provinces (Romanow, 2002). In response to this policy problem, some experts have long argued for a single national drug plan and formulary as well as a single agency to regulate pharmaceutical pricing. However, such an approach is challenged by two opposing imperatives: that of provincial governments, especially Quebec, which wish to retain control over provincial drug policies including prescription drug plans, and that of the federal government, which has resisted assuming the financial burden and future fiscal risk of a federally financed and administered pharmaceutical coverage programme (Marchildon, 2007).

With the exception of Quebec, governments agreed to allow CADTH to establish a pan-Canadian process to review the clinical and cost-effectiveness of new prescription drugs the CDR, which began in 2003. However, the CDR makes only recommendations, and provincial governments ultimately decide whether or not to consider CDR analyses in determining whether or not to include specific pharmaceuticals in their respective formularies. In 2004, as part of the *10-Year Plan to Strengthen Health Care* signed by first ministers, all P/T governments, except for Quebec, established a task force of ministers of health to develop and implement a "National Pharmaceuticals Strategy" that encompassed the following nine action items (CICS, 2004):

- in response to ongoing concerns about the financial insecurity caused by poor and inconsistent coverage of expensive drugs (Phillips, 2009), to develop, assess and cost the options for catastrophic coverage;
- establish a common national drug formulary for participating jurisdictions based on safety and cost-effectiveness;
- accelerate access to breakthrough drugs for unmet health needs through improvement to the federal drug approval process;
- strengthen evaluation of drug safety and effectiveness;
- pursue purchasing strategies to obtain best prices for Canadians for drugs and vaccines;
- enhance action to influence the prescribing behaviour of health care professionals so that drugs are used only when needed and the right drug is used for the right problem;
- broaden the practice of e-prescribing through accelerated development and deployment of EHRs;
- accelerate access to non-patented drugs and achieve international parity on prices of generic drugs; and

- enhance analysis of cost drivers and cost-effectiveness, including best practices, in public drug plan policies.

Although the ministerial committee made incremental progress, work on the nine reform items had largely come to a halt by the end of the decade. This was due in part to changes in federal and provincial government administrations in the intervening years, and it leaves a large policy vacuum that remains to be addressed in the future (HCC, 2009).

5.7 Rehabilitation/intermediate care

Inpatient rehabilitation services provided in hospitals and specialized rehabilitation facilities are deemed medically necessary services and are available without charge to Canadians. Inpatient rehabilitation tends to focus on orthopaedics (immediately following hip and knee replacement surgery), stroke, brain dysfunction, limb amputation and spinal cord injury, with almost two-thirds (63%) involving orthopaedic and post-stroke rehabilitation (CIHI, 2008a). Public coverage, including workers' compensation for outpatient rehabilitation services, varies by province and territory, and PHI coverage and OOP payments are common (Landry et al., 2008; Landry, Raman & Al-Hamdan, 2010). These outpatient services are generally provided in clinics or workplaces directed by physiotherapists or occupational therapists.

5.8 Long-term care

This section focuses on long-term care provision for older adults as well as individuals of any age with physical disabilities, chronic diseases or learning disabilities. LTC can be provided in facility-based institutions or in the community through home care and other support services. Care for acute and chronic mental health disorders are discussed in section 5.11. Since long-term care is not considered an insured service under the Canada Health Act, public policies, subsidies, programmes and regulatory regimes for long-term care vary among the provinces and territories (Chan & Kenny, 2002; Berta et al., 2006; Hirdes, 2002).

There is a variety of facility-based long-term care in Canada, ranging from residential care with some assisted living services to chronic care facilities – which used to be called nursing homes – with 24-hour a day nursing supervision.

Most residential care is privately funded whereas most high-acuity long-term care providing 24-hour a day nursing supervision is publicly funded by the provincial and territorial governments. long-term care facilities face different provincial and territorial regimes in terms of licensing and quality control as well as accreditation requirements. Ownership also varies considerably across the country (Berta et al., 2006). In some provinces, a majority of publicly funded long-term care beds are in profit-making facilities: for example, in Ontario, 60% of publicly-funded beds are in profit-making facilities (Berta, Laporte & Valdamanis, 2005). In other provinces, a majority of publicly funded long-term care beds are in not-for-profit facilities, owned either by the provincial government and regional health authorities or by community-based or faith-based organizations; for example, in British Columbia, 70% of publicly-funded long-term care beds are in non-profit-making facilities (McGrail et al., 2007). In all cases, the non-profit-making facilities tend to be larger with higher direct care staffing levels because their residents' needs tend to be more complex, requiring higher levels of care (Berta et al., 2006). While there is some evidence that better patient outcomes are associated with non-profit-making long-term care facilities compared with profit-making homes, more research is needed to test this association (McGrail et al., 2007).

In the more highly integrated provincial and territorial health systems, home-based care can be a cost-effective alternative to facility-based care. Moreover, increases in publicly funded home care in Canada have been shown to reduce the use of hospital services, reduce reliance on informal caregivers and increase self-perceived levels of health status (Stabile, Laporte & Coyte, 2006; Hollander et al., 2009). Although the percentage, and basic profile, of Canadians receiving publicly subsidized home care changed little between the mid-1990s and the mid-2000s (Table 5.2), there is evidence that the needs of those receiving home care have grown in acuity. For example, while 8% of home-care recipients were incontinent in 1994–1995, the proportion more than doubled to 17% by 2003 (Wilkins, 2006).

Table 5.2
Characteristics of recipients of government-subsidized home care in Canada, 1994–1995 and 2003

	1994–95	2003
Canadian population receiving subsidized home care, 18 and over (%)	2.5	2.7
Female (%)	32.7	34.6
Social assistance as main source of income (%)	38.9	33.8
Average number of days in hospital in past year	13.4	8.6
Average age in years	64.9	62.0

Source: Wilkins (2006).

Similar to other high-income countries, older frail Canadians are the recipients of most facility- and home-based long-term care. In most provinces, long-term care has increasingly been integrated into geographically-based health care system through RHAs, and provincial ministries of health generally have a division responsible for long-term care. There are also a number of private services and accommodation, particularly in larger urban centres, that can be purchased by older Canadians and their families.

5.9 Services for informal carers

Each province and territory has its own policies and programmes for informal caregivers generally as part of the package of home care services and benefits provided by the particular P/T government. Since 2002, the federal government has provided tax credits for eligible caregivers. In response to the work completed by the national Secretariat on Palliative and End-of-Life Care (2001–2007), the Government of Canada introduced the Compassionate Care Benefit, which offers workers six weeks paid leave from their employment to support family members who are in the final six months of life. The Compassionate Care Benefit is part of the Employment Insurance Programme and is, therefore, not available to non-standard employees and the self-employed.[2]

Consequently, the Compassionate Care Benefit is limited in its support of unpaid carers (Flagler & Dong, 2010; Williams et al., 2011). Recent estimates of the economic value of unpaid caregivers reveal the extent to which home-based long-term care depends on volunteerism (Hollander, Guiping & Chappell, 2009). However, researchers as well as caregiver advocacy groups have questioned the

[2] Although some of these benefits have recently been extended to the self-employed on a voluntary basis, enrolment has been low because only a tiny percentage of the self-employed have been willing to pay the premiums.

sustainability of this policy. One research study concluded that the higher the proportion of non-kin, male and geographically distant members that make up a given patient's informal care network, the less sustainable the care (Fast et al., 2004). In some cases, informal caregiving, may be inadequate. There also appears to be an urban–rural divide in the support of informal caregivers with many more programmes in place for urban caregivers (Crosato & Leipert, 2006). There are also major differences in terms of the quality of home-support services more generally (Sims-Gould & Martin-Matthews, 2010).

5.10 Palliative care

Since the terms "hospice care" and "palliative care" are used interchangeably in Canada despite their different historical meanings (Syme & Bruce, 2009), the term "palliative care" as used here includes both forms of care. Wright et al. (2008) have demonstrated that there is a positive correlation between income as well as human development, as measured by the United Nations' Human Development Index (HDI), and the availability of palliative care services across countries. As such, Canada is similar to high-income and high-HDI countries in the OECD in terms of the provision and integration of palliative care services. Similar to the overall public–private split in the funding of health care, slightly more than 70% of palliative care services are publicly funded through F/P/T health plans (Dumont et al., 2009).[3]

The level of public funding is due in part to the fact that most palliative care in Canada is provided to patients dying of cancer, who, in turn, receive a substantial amount of end-of-life care in hospital, despite in some cases the preference for home-based palliative care (Leeb, Morris & Kasman, 2005; Widger et al., 2007). However, in recent years, there has been a dramatic shift in the location of end-of-life care. In the period 1994–2004, the proportion of Canadians dying in hospital dropped from 77.7% to 60.6% while those dying in long-term care facilities rose from 3% to 9.9% and those dying at home rose from 19.3% to 29.5% (Wilson et al., 2008).

Since it was founded in 1991, the Canadian Hospice Palliative Care Association (CHPCA), a charitable non-profit-making organization, has been a consistent advocate for improving access to palliative care outside hospitals, and for the setting of national norms and practice guidelines for outpatient palliative care (Canadian Hospice Palliative Care Association, 2002). This is due in part

[3] The federal government is mentioned in this context because Veterans Affairs Canada offers palliative care services to eligible veterans of the Canadian Armed Forces.

to the enormous differences in the nature of these services across Canada, as illustrated for home-based palliative care in Table 5.3. In addition, the Senate of Canada has both raised awareness of palliative care and recommended a pan-Canadian strategy for a more consistent, comprehensive and integrated system of palliative care (Senate of Canada, 2010).

Table 5.3
Home-based palliative care services by jurisdiction in Canada, 2008

Province or territory	24/7 access to nursing–personal care services	24/7 access to case management services	Protocol for timely referrals	Wait time tracking	Policy for team-based care	Inter-professional education	Support for research
British Columbia	*	–	–	–	*	–	–
Alberta	*	–	–	–	*	*	*
Saskatchewan	–	*	*	–	*	–	–
Manitoba	*	–	*	–	*	*	*
Ontario	*	*	*	*	–	*	*
New Brunswick	*	–	*	*	*	–	–
Nova Scotia	*	–	–	–	–	–	–
Prince Edward Island	–	–	*	–	*	*	*
Newfoundland and Labrador	–	*	*	–	*	*	*
Nunavut	–	–	*	*	*	*	*
Northwest Territories	–	–	–	*	–	–	–
Yukon	–	–	*	–	*	*	*

Source: Derived from Quality End-of-Life Coalition of Canada (2008).
Note: Quebec did not participate in the survey.

The majority of larger hospitals in Canada have palliative care units, a development that originated with the division of cancer treatment into curative and palliative in the 1970s. While hospital-based end-of-life care is relatively consistent in Canada, there are important differences in terms of home-based palliative care services funded and administered by provincial and territorial governments (Quality End-of-Life Coalition of Canada, 2008). There is also considerable variety in palliative care policies and programmes across the country (Williams et al., 2010).

5.11 Mental health care

Over the past half-century, mental health care for individuals with severe and chronic mental illness has evolved from an emphasis on large psychiatric hospitals, in which patients resided for very long periods of time, to more episodic treatment in the psychiatric wings of hospitals and outpatient care involving prescription drug therapies. The "deinstitutionalization" that occurred in the 1960s and early 1970s was precipitated by changing professional therapies in conjunction with the introduction of new pharmaceutical therapies (Sealy & Whitehead, 2004; Dyck, 2011).

For historical reasons, some mental health services, particularly those not provided in hospitals or by physicians, have never been included as fully insured services under the CHA. The policy legacies associated with the development of universal medicare in Canada included an emphasis on hospital-based treatment and a privileged position for doctors – family physicians and psychiatrists – over other mental health care providers (Mulvale, Abelson & Goering, 2007). For example, the services provided by psychologists are largely private and paid for through PHI as part of employment benefit packages or OOP payments (Romanow & Marchildon, 2003).

As a consequence, in part, of this policy legacy, family physicians provide the majority of primary mental health services in Canada. The results of a recent large sample survey of family physicians in Saskatchewan revealed that 80% of the respondents saw a least six patients a week with mental health problems, while one-quarter of these same physicians saw more than 20 patients with mental health conditions a week. A large number of the family physicians were frustrated with the quality of the services they rendered to their patients. Furthermore, 60% of these family physicians co-managed their patients' mental health problems with other professions, and they were particularly dissatisfied with the co-management with psychiatrists (Clatney, MacDonald & Shah, 2008).

Like almost all other OECD countries, Canada's mental health outcomes in term of mental and behavioural disorders has not improved appreciably since the implementation of deinstitutionalization (OECD, 2008). In 2006, the Standing Senate Committee on Social Affairs, Science and Technology recommended that a national commission be established to develop a pan-Canadian policy for mental health care and addictions (Senate of Canada, 2006). One year later, the Mental Health Commission of Canada was established by the federal government with the endorsement of all provinces and territories except for Quebec. In 2012, after extensive consultations with governmental and nongovernmental stakeholders, the Commission released its first major report setting out a mental health strategy (MHCC, 2009, MHCC, 2012).

Due to data limitations, there are few studies that compare the quality and volume of mental health care in Canada with other countries. In their study comparing Canada with Australia, Tempier et al. (2009) found a much higher level of anxiety disorders in the Canadian population (4.6%) relative to the Australian population (2.7%), although the rate of alcohol and drug dependence was somewhat lower. Despite similarities in the levels and availability of mental health providers, mental health consultations were lower in Canada (51.3%) relative to Australia (64.6%).

5.12 Dental care

Almost all dental health services are delivered by independent practitioners operating their own practices. Payment for these services is through PHI or direct OOP payment. If a provincial or territorial resident is receiving social assistance, then a portion or all of the costs for personal dental services may be covered by the provincial or territorial government. Similarly, if an individual is an eligible First Nation or Inuit, then a portion or all of the costs will be covered by the federal government through the "non-insured health benefits" programme. Almost 54% of all private-funded dental care is funded through PHI, the majority of which is through employment-based benefit plans (Hurley & Guindon, 2008). The remaining amount is funded directly by OOP payments.

Unlike most high-income countries, Canada provides a very low level of public subsidies to access dental care. Currently, 95% of all dental services are funded privately, a level that is similar to the United States, Spain and Portugal, the only other wealthy countries with such high levels of private finance for dental services (Grignon et al., 2010). This degree of dependence on private funding, in the absence of other barriers to access, has produced high levels of inequalities in terms of dental care (Leake & Birch, 2008; Wallace & MacEntee, 2012). These inequalities are directly linked to the fact that lower income Canadians visit dentists less often due to cost (Health Canada, 2010).

In order to address these inequities, a few targeted oral health and dental service programmes have been initiated by governments. The first provincial programme of this type, launched by the Government of Saskatchewan in the 1970s, targeted school children. Utilizing dental nurses and dental para-professionals, the Saskatchewan Health Dental Program proved to be highly effective but was disbanded within a decade (Wolfson, 1997). This was followed by a similar programme in Manitoba targeting rural children but it too was eventually discontinued by a subsequent administration (Marchildon, 2011). Ontario has the CINOT (Children in Need of Treatment Program) as well as Health Smiles Ontario, a low-income programme launched in 2010

(Ito, 2011). As mentioned above, the federal government funds the largest targeted programme in Canada by providing dental care coverage under the "non-insured health benefits" programme.

5.13 Complementary and alternative medicine

CAM embraces entire non-Western systems of medicine, such as traditional Chinese medicine and Aboriginal healing, as well as specific medicines and therapies such as herbalism, relaxation therapy and reflexology. Jonas & Levin (1999) have catalogued some 4000 different CAM practices including homeopathy, chiropractic and therapeutic massage. Although these practices vary considerably, most CAM therapies share at least four common characteristics (Smith & Simpson, 2003):

- they are presumed to work in conjunction with the body's own self-healing mechanisms;
- they are "holistic" in the sense that they treat the whole person;
- they try to involve the individual as an active participant in the healing process; and
- they focus on disease prevention and well-being as much as treatment.

As is the case in most OECD countries, Canadians have shown increasing interest in CAM. The rate of growth of at least some classes of alternative practitioner has outstripped the rate of growth in mainstream health care providers (Clarke, 2004). At the same time, the response of the established health care professions to emerging CAM practitioners ranges from acceptance to scepticism and even hostility (Kelner et al., 2004; Nahas & Balla, 2011). Some CAM groups, including naturopaths, traditional Chinese medicine acupuncturists and homeopaths have responded to these challenges by pursuing further professionalization including self-regulation (Welsh et al., 2004; Gilmour et al., 2002).

Since 2004, natural health products have been regulated by Health Canada's Natural Health Product Directorate. Health Canada defines health products as products containing only those ingredients listed on Schedule 1 of the Food and Drugs Act's Natural Health Products Regulations (e.g. plant or plant material, alga, bacterium, fungus, mineral, amino acid and vitamin), homeopathic medicines or traditional medicines, and it excludes those products containing ingredients listed on Schedule 2 (e.g. tobacco, controlled drugs or substances, and antibiotics prepared from alga, bacterium or fungus). Natural health products are sold in dosage form and are designed for: use in the diagnosis, treatment, mitigation or prevention of a disease, disorder or abnormal physical state or its symptoms in humans; to maintain or promote health; to restore or correct human health function; to restore or correct organic functions in humans; or to modify organic functions in humans in a manner that maintains or promotes health. Based on a Statistics Canada survey completed in 2007, there were 290 specialist health product firms in Canada selling tens of thousands of natural health products and generating C$1.7 billion in revenues (Cinnamon, 2009).

5.14 Health services for Aboriginal Canadians

The term "Aboriginal Canadians" includes First Nations, Inuit and Métis residents, a reference to the descendants of peoples who lived in the geographical expanses now called Canada before European settlement. Provincial and territorial governments are responsible for providing all their residents, including Aboriginal Canadians, with insured services under the Canada Health Act. The federal government funds and administers nursing stations, health promotion/disease prevention programmes and public health services on First Nation reserves and in Inuit communities and also provides on-reserve primary care and emergency care services in remote and isolated areas where P/T insured services are not available. In addition, the federal government provides roughly 846 000 eligible First Nations and Inuit with non-insured health benefits (see section 2.3.2).

Historically, government efforts to target the health needs of Aboriginal Canadians have achieved limited success. For example, in the case of dental health, federally funded coverage of dental services for eligible First Nations and Inuit under the "non-insured health benefits" programme seems to have had a limited impact on reducing disparities between Aboriginal and non-Aboriginal Canadians (Lawrence et al., 2009; Grignon et al., 2010).

As a consequence of these persistent disparities, Aboriginal organizations and leaders have argued for greater control over the funding and delivery of health services. Since the 1990s, a series of health-funding transfer agreements between the federal government and eligible First Nations and Inuit organizations has permitted a greater degree of Aboriginal control, particularly in areas of primary health care (Lavoie, 2004). Such initiatives have spurred an Aboriginal health movement advocating a more uniquely Aboriginal philosophy to health and health care. In the same vein, the National Aboriginal Health Organization (NAHO) was established in 2000 with a mandate to improve the health of First Nation, Inuit and Métis individuals, families and communities.[4] According to Lemchuk-Favel & Jock (2004), the strengths of the Aboriginal health movement, beyond the potential benefits of self-empowerment and control, includes holistic healing that takes a culturally distinct approach to primary health care with an emphasis on the synergies produced by combining indigenous health and medicines with more conventional health approaches.

[4] NAHO was officially closed in June 2012 following cuts in the federal governments budget of 2012.

6. Principal health reforms

Since 2005, when the first edition of this study was published (Marchildon, 2005), there have been no major pan-Canadian health reform initiatives. However, individual provincial and territorial ministries of health have concentrated on two categories of reform, one involving the reorganization or fine tuning of their regional health systems, and the second linked to improving the quality and timeliness of – and patient experience with – primary, acute and chronic care.

The main purpose of regionalization was to gain the benefits of vertical integration by managing facilities and providers across a broad continuum of health services, in particular to improve the coordination of "downstream" curative services with more "upstream" public health and illness prevention services and interventions. In the last ten years, in an attempt to capture economies of scale and scope in service delivery as well as reduce infrastructure costs, there has been a trend to greater centralization, with provincial ministries of health reducing the number of RHAs (see Table 2.3). Two provinces, Alberta and Prince Edward Island, now have a single RHA responsible for coordinating all acute and long-term care services (but not primary care) in their respective provinces.

Influenced chiefly by quality improvement initiatives in the United States and the United Kingdom, provincial ministries of health established institutions and mechanisms to improve the quality, safety, timeliness and responsiveness of health services. Six provinces established health quality councils to accelerate quality improvement initiatives. Two provincial governments also launched patient-centred initiatives aimed at improving the experience of both patients and caregivers. Most ministries and RHAs also implemented some aspects of performance measurement in an effort to improve outcomes and processes. Patient dissatisfaction with long waiting times in hospital EDs and for certain types of elective surgery such as joint replacements has triggered efforts in all provinces to better manage and reduce waiting times.

In contrast, there has been more limited progress on the intergovernmental front since the first ministers' *10-Year Plan to Strengthen Health Care* (CICS, 2004). Following that meeting, provincial and territorial governments used additional federal cash transfers to shorten waiting times in priority areas, reinvigorate primary care reform and provide additional coverage for home care services that could be substituted for hospital care. While a number of provincial and territorial governments introduced some form of catastrophic drug coverage for their own residents, they achieved very little in forging a pan-Canadian approach to prescription drug coverage and management.

6.1 Analysis of recent reforms

The modern era of Canadian health care reform began in the late 1980s and early 1990s after the passage of the Canada Health Act (1984). This federal law locked in place a pattern of universal coverage that had originally been established through the Hospital Insurance and Diagnostic Services Act (1957) and the Medical Care Act (1966). By withdrawing transfer funding from those jurisdictions permitting user fees and extra billing on a dollar-for-dollar basis, and then returning most of the nearly C$250 million originally withdrawn after the offending provinces had eliminated user fees and extra billing, the federal government entrenched the principle of first dollar coverage.

Since universal coverage remained limited to medically necessary hospital and physician services – with no sustained effort to expand this basket of universally covered services – this "narrow but deep" coverage has remained the policy status quo ever since in Canada. At the same time, the law discouraged governments from reducing universal coverage for health care despite major cuts in public spending in response to decades of deficit-spending and a slowing economy in the early to mid-1990s. Conversely, when the economy improved and governments benefited from a fiscal bonus because of reduced payments on the debt, they chose not to increase universal coverage even marginally despite the recommendations of a Royal Commission (Romanow, 2002) and a Senate Committee (Senate of Canada 2002). As a consequence, there have been no major changes to the universal basket of health services since medicare was introduced.

In what follows, more recent and incremental health reforms have been separated into two movements, one driven by the desire for greater coordination and integration through structural reorganization, and the second motivated by concerns about quality of care. In the first set of reforms, governments across

Canada, encouraged by policy experts and numerous commission reports, attempted to exert some managerial control over what had been a passive payment system. However, rationalization and the squeezing of global health budgets in the 1990s also created the perception that services had deteriorated. In response to voter dissatisfaction, governments substantially increased spending on health services. Since 2000, accompanied by a large increase in spending by Canadian governments, reforms have focused on improving the quality and timeliness of health services.

During the 1990s, most provincial governments – in the words of one deputy minister of health – were racing two horses simultaneously: a "black horse" of cost-cutting through health facility and human resource rationalization and a "white horse" of health reform to improve both quality and access through a more managed integration of services across the health continuum, as well as a rebalancing from illness care to "wellness" services (Adams, 2001). Cost-cutting was accomplished, at least in part, through reducing the number of hospital beds and health providers. In response to the reduction in the demand for hospital care, spurred by new medical technologies that reduced the length of stay, some hospitals were closed, others converted into long-term care facilities or wellness centres, and still others were consolidated into larger units.

In every province, service delivery was rationalized in one form or another in response to restrictive health budgets. In Ontario, it was achieved through an arm's length commission responsible for recommending and implementing hospital consolidation (Sinclair, Rochon & Leatt, 2005) while in a number of other provinces, it was achieved through RHAs. However, the main purpose of regionalization was to gain the benefits of vertical integration: that is, managing facilities and providers across the continuum of care in a single administrative organization capable of improving the coordination of curative and preventative services for individual patients as well as population-level interventions (Marchildon, 2006; Axelsson, Marchildon & Repullo-Labrador, 2007). This structural reform was central to the recommendations of arm's length commissions and task forces that delivered their reports to the Governments of Quebec (1988), Nova Scotia (1989), Alberta (1989), Ontario (1990), Saskatchewan (1990) and British Columbia (1991), helping create a structural reform momentum in the 1990s (Mhatre & Deber, 1992).

There remains considerable debate concerning regionalization as a reform. In addition, despite major improvements in data collection at the RHA level by the CIHI, as of 2011 there had not been a systematic and comparative assessment as to whether this structural reform has achieved its main health policy objectives, including shifting more resources from curative care to illness prevention and health promotion interventions and initiatives at both the individual and population health level.

Influenced by the quality improvement movements and initiatives in the United States and the United Kingdom, ministries of health in Canada also established institutions and mechanisms to improve the quality, safety, timeliness and client-responsiveness of health services. Six provincial governments set up quality councils to work with health organizations and providers to provide higher-quality care, reduce the rate of medical errors and improve both efficiency and health care outcomes. Most ministries and RHAs use at least some indicators and measures to identify poor performance and improve both processes and outcomes. At the pan-Canadian level, the Health Council of Canada identifies best practices and evaluates performance in key health reform areas and disseminates the results to all governments as well as the general public.

By the mid- to late 1990s, governments were beginning to invest time and resources in their health information, research and data management infrastructures. In 1994, the federal and provincial governments established the CIHI to hold, improve, use and disseminate administrative data as part of a larger effort by governments to better understand and evaluate their respective health systems. CIHI was initially a consolidation of activities from Statistics Canada, health information programmes from Health Canada, the Hospital Medical Records Institute and the Management Information Systems group. In partnership with Statistics Canada, CIHI has grown into one of the world's premier national health information repositories, with extensive databases on health spending, services, infrastructure and human resources.

These improvements in the collection, organization and dissemination of health system data were spurred by the recommendations of arm's length commissions and ministerial task forces, including major reports for provincial governments in Ontario (2000), Quebec (2000), Saskatchewan (2001) and Alberta (2001) as well as for the federal government (Romanow 2002; Senate of Canada, 2002). At the same time, health ministries in Canada have been less willing than other OECD health ministries to use performance indicators as a tool in managing the delivery organizations in their respective health systems. They have been reluctant to create the intergovernmental processes and institutions to facilitate systematic comparisons of the performance across provincial health systems, including the establishment of voluntary (intergovernmental) forms of performance benchmarking (Fenna, 2010; Fafard, 2012).

Following the Romanow Royal Commission's recommendations of 2002, F/P/T first ministers met to decide which commission recommendations could be implemented. In the resulting *First Ministers' Accord on Health Care Renewal,* they focused on re-igniting primary care reform, improving catastrophic drug coverage, facilitating greater substitution of home care services for hospital-based services and accelerating the adoption of EHRs (CICS, 2003).

In 2004, F/P/T first ministers negotiated *A 10-Year Plan to Strengthen Health Care,* the most significant intergovernmental health accord reached in the last decade. In addition to increasing the level of the Canada Health Transfer, the 10-Year Plan also guaranteed that the federal government would increase federal health transfers to the provinces and territories by 6% per year for the following decade. In return for this generous funding, the provincial and territorial governments agreed on the proposed plan's key policy priorities, including waiting times, home care and pharmaceutical policy. While some governments have made progress in one or more of these areas, as reviewed below, the collaborative or pan-Canadian aspect of these efforts especially those aimed at transformative changes, were not realised (Senate of Canada, 2012).

The 10-Year Plan was facilitated by a federal Wait Time Reduction Fund (C$5.5 billion over 10 years) to assist provinces in meeting their waiting time targets in five priority areas – cancer, cardiac, sight restoration, joint replacement and diagnostic imaging. Provincial and territorial governments worked with the CIHI to establish benchmarks for every priority area except diagnostic imaging.[1] All provinces provide CIHI with comparable waiting times data, and all provinces,[2] with the exceptions of Manitoba and Newfoundland and Labrador, have set targets based on individually established benchmarks (Fafard, 2012). In addition, all provinces inform their residents about waiting times in these priority areas. Overall, they have made progress in managing and reducing surgical and diagnostic waiting times since 2004. While there remains considerable variation across provinces, most Canadians receive these priority procedures within the benchmarks set by the provinces (CIHI, 2012b).

1 According to the majority of participants, there was insufficient evidence on the appropriate waiting times for diagnostic imaging.

2 Since patients living in the territories are usually referred to hospitals in the provinces for elective surgeries, the three territories are excluded in the remainder of the discussion on waiting times.

Since 2004, provincial governments have had very mixed results in effecting the reforms necessary to meet the waiting time targets despite the influx of extra federal funding.

In the 10-Year Plan, governments agreed to extend first-dollar coverage for targeted home care services in three areas: (1) two weeks of acute home care after release from hospital; (2) two weeks of acute mental health home care; and (3) end-of-life home care. It appears that most provinces now provide coverage for these limited services, although considerable provincial and territorial variability for other home care services remains the rule (Canadian Healthcare Association, 2009).

Progress on primary care was also identified as a policy priority under the 10-Year Plan. All governments agreed to provide at least 50% of their respective populations with (24-hour, 7-day-a-week) access to multidisciplinary primary care teams by 2011, a major commitment given the fact that the vast majority of primary care was still being provided by physicians in 2004. While it has not yet been calculated whether any jurisdiction has reached the 24/7 target, it does appear that approximately three-quarters of family physicians are now working in multi-professional practices (Hutchison et al., 2011).

With the exception of the Government of Quebec, which declared that it would not abandon or change its provincial prescription drug plan, the 2004 accord also committed P/T governments to work with the federal government on what became known as the National Pharmaceuticals Strategy. Under the direction of F/P/T health ministers, this initiative was to create a pan-Canadian system of prescription drug coverage and pricing policy. However, despite some early progress, the National Pharmaceuticals Strategy eventually died due to lack of interest among the participating governments, one of the more notable failures of the 10-Year Plan (HCC, 2009; MacKinnon & Ip, 2009). While a number of provincial governments have introduced catastrophic drug coverage on their own, this has sometimes come at the price of rolling back categorical coverage for older Canadians, and it is unclear whether these changes have produced an overall improvement in financial protection (Daw & Morgan, 2012).

6.2 Future developments

The 10-Year Plan ends in the fiscal year 2013–2014. Debate concerning the future of the federal role and its funding commitments to the provinces and territories featured prominently in the 2011 federal election. Months after the election – in December 2011 – the federal government announced its decision on the future of the Canada Health Transfer, a unilateral decision in an area that has been subject to considerable intergovernmental discussion in recent years. For this reason, it was met with considerable surprise by provincial and territorial governments as well as the media. One of the most important substantive changes to the Canada Health Transfer will be the termination of a regional equalization component that benefited less wealthy provinces. After 2014, provincial shares of the transfer will be distributed on a pure per capita basis. While the federal government has agreed to continue to increase the transfer by 6% for an additional three years post-2014, after 2016–2017, any increases in the Canada Health Transfer will be tied to the rate of the country's economic growth, with a minimum floor of 3%. At the same time, the federal government announced it would no longer use its spending power to encourage or set health system goals. Instead, it would look to the provincial governments to establish their own health reform priorities and objectives.

During the past decade, the buoyant Canadian economy and the positive fiscal position of the federal and provincial governments produced a fiscal dividend much of which was used for health care and the reduction of taxes. With the slowing of the economy since 2008, this fiscal dividend is disappearing, and both orders of government face harder budget constraints and more difficult choices in terms of health spending. Similar to what occurred in the early to mid-1990s (Tuohy, 2002), this is likely not only to put pressure on achieving more rapid progress on existing health reforms but may also precipitate new health reforms aimed at increasing value for money.

7. Assessment of the health system

In assessing performance, the Canadian health system has been effective in financially protecting Canadians against high-cost hospital and physician services. At the same time, the narrow scope of universal services covered under medicare has produced important gaps in coverage. With regard to prescription drugs and dental care, for example, depending on employment and province or territory of residence, these gaps are filled by PHI and, at least for drug therapies, by provincial plans that target seniors and the very poor. Where public coverage of drugs and dental care does not fill in the cracks left by private coverage, equitable access is a major challenge. Since the majority of funding for health care comes from general tax revenues of the F/P/T governments, and the revenue sources range from progressive to proportionate, there is equity in financing. However, to the extent that financing is OOP and through employment-based insurance benefits that are associated with better-paid jobs, there is less equity in financing.

There are disparities in terms of access to health care but, outside a few areas such as dental care and mental health care, they do not appear to be large. For example, there appears to be a pro-poor bias in terms of primary care use but a pro-rich bias in the use of specialist physician services, but the gap in both cases is not large. Canada's east–west economic gradient, with less wealthy provinces in the east and more wealthy provinces in the west, is systematically addressed through equalization payments from federal revenue sources made to "have-not" provinces to ensure they have the revenues necessary to provide comparable levels of public services including health care without resorting to prohibitively high tax rates.

While Canadians are generally satisfied with the financial protection offered by medicare in particular, they are less satisfied with other aspects determining access. In particular, starting in the 1990s, they became dissatisfied with access to physicians and crowded emergency departments in hospitals as well as lengthening waiting times for non-urgent surgery. In a 2010 survey of patients by the Commonwealth Fund, for example, Canada ranked behind Australia, France, Sweden, the United Kingdom and the United States in terms of patient experience of waiting times for physician care and non-urgent surgery (HCC, 2011b). Using more objective indicators of health system performance such as amenable mortality, however, Canadian health system performance is more positive, with much better outcomes than the United Kingdom and the United States, although not quite as good as Australia, Sweden and France. Canadian performance on an index of health care quality indicators has also improved over the past decade as provincial governments, assisted by health quality councils and other organizations, more systemically implement quality improvement measures. Finally, governments, health care organizations and providers are making more efforts to improve the overall patient experience.

7.1 Stated objectives of the health system

Based on the history of medicare supported by provincial and territorial medicare laws as well as the Canada Health Act, Canadians expect to continue receiving universal access to medically necessary hospital and physician services without any direct charges. This expectation – which is often perceived as a basic right by Canadians – highlights the role of both orders of government in financially protecting individuals in the event that health care is needed. It also implies that Canadians should have equitable access to medically necessary services, an assumption that is reflected in the criteria of universality and accessibility in the Canada Health Act and the restatement of these principles in provincial and territorial medicare laws. However, health care involves much more than medicare, and there is less financial protection and equity of access when it comes to prescription drugs, long-term care, dental care and vision care.

Although results vary depending on the sector in question, in general, health and health service outcomes, including quality, based on a series of measures are reasonably good in Canada. However, patient satisfaction ratings are not as good, at least when compared with selected OECD countries. While this is, no doubt, a consequence of a number of factors, dissatisfaction with long waiting times is probably one of the most important – if not the most important – contributing factors. Another may be the historic lack of transparency and accountability in Canadian health care, something that governments are now addressing by providing more information on waiting lists, patient navigation, benefits and quality, as well as the reform and performance objectives of provincial ministries of health, RHAs and other health care organizations.

7.2 Financial protection and equity in financing

7.2.1 Financial protection

Financial protection measures the extent to which individuals are protected from the financial consequences of illness. Three factors underpin the need for financial protection: uncertainty about the need for health care due to the unpredictability of the timing and severity of illness; the high cost of most interventions and treatments; and the potential loss of earnings due to ill health.

Historically, financial protection was the key motivation behind the introduction of universal medicare in Canada. Although coverage is deep (no user fees), the scope of medicare is narrow, limited as it is to hospital and physician services. As a result, there continues to be a debate as to whether financial protection is adequate for pharmaceuticals, dental care and other sectors and services not included in medicare.

Table 7.1 focuses on the mix of OOP and PHI coverage in non-medicare sectors and services. When it comes to prescription drugs, PHI constitutes as important a source of coverage as public coverage plans. In the 1990s, many argued in favour of a national, universal pharmacare programme that would

Table 7.1
OOP spending relative to private health insurance coverage for non-medicare services, amount (C$ billions) and % of total health care spending in Canada, 2008

	OOP spending ($C billions)	% of health spending in category	PHI spending ($C billions)	% of health spending in category
Prescription drugs	4.2	17.8	8.5	36.1
Over-the-counter drugs and personal health supplies	4.5	100.0	0.0	0.0
Dental care	5.2	44.4	6.0	51.0
Professionals other than physicians providing medicare	4.3	64.3	1.6	24.1
Institutions other than hospitals	4.9	28.5	0.0	0.0

Sources: CIHI (2010b); Hurley & Guindon (2011).

provide first-dollar coverage. By the 2000s, largely for cost reasons, this had shifted to various proposals for a more targeted, catastrophic drug programme with last-dollar coverage. Even though pan-Canadian policy efforts have failed, the majority of provinces have introduced catastrophic coverage for prescription drugs in the last decade. However, due to high levels of patient cost-sharing as well as the reduction in coverage for older Canadians in some provinces, these changes have not necessarily increased overall coverage (Daw & Morgan, 2012).

There is virtually no public coverage for dental care. While provincial governments have, occasionally, provided targeted coverage for children's dental care, there has been no sustained momentum for either universal coverage on a pan-Canadian basis or in individual provinces (Marchildon, 2011).

Almost two-thirds of the cost of non-physician services provided by most other health care professionals are paid through OOP payments. A further 25% of the cost is covered through PHI and a miniscule percentage through the public purse. These professionals include dentists, psychologists, chiropractors, optometrists, physiotherapists and occupational therapists among others. Although some of these groups have occasionally been successful in obtaining some public coverage for their services, this coverage varies considerably across provinces and territories.

In Canada, there is very little PHI coverage for institutional long-term care. However, every province and territory provides targeted subsidies for individuals requiring more intensive long-term care and this is reflected in the fact that OOP payments account for less than one-third of the total outlay in this category. To date, there has been no concerted policy effort to address the lack of financial protection for long-term care in part because of the means-tested subsidies offered by all provincial and territorial governments.

7.2.2 Equity in financing

Equity in financing is determined by the extent to which individual sources of health financing are progressive, proportional or regressive. A health-financing source is progressive if the proportion of income an individual pays increases with income. A financing source is regressive if the proportion of income an individual pays decreases. The financing source is proportionate if the proportion of income an individual pays remains the same at all income levels. The more progressive the health-financing system, the greater the equity in financing.

As discussed in Chapter 3, OOP payments made up 15% of revenues and PHI a further 13% of revenues for all health spending in Canada in 2009, almost all of which stems from the benefit packages in group-based employment plans. Such benefits are generally restricted to higher-wage and higher-salary permanent jobs, whereas the working poor are often in low-paid, temporary or seasonal jobs, precisely the type of employment that does not come with PHI benefits (Hurley & Guindon, 2008). By health sector, dental care provides one of the most extreme examples of reliance on private funding. In Canada, 95% of all financing for dental care comes from either OOP or PHI sources, a figure considerably higher than in almost all high-income OECD countries.

Compared with PHI and OOP funding sources, general tax revenues are more equitable, involving some income redistribution from higher-income households to lower-income households. The extent of this redistribution depends on the overall degree of progressivity of the general tax system. As reviewed in Chapter 3, a number of revenue sources make up the general revenue funds of governments in Canada. Although the largest source is income tax – a progressive source of taxation – other taxes, including consumption taxes, tend to be regressive, making it difficult to assess the progressivity of the tax system as a whole. While tax systems are often perceived to be progressive, the reality depends on the relative mix and design of taxes that make up the basket of the general revenue funds of an individual government – federal, provincial or territorial.

In her analysis of the equity of health financing in British Columbia, McGrail (2007) found that the mix and incidence of taxes actually resulted in a health-financing system that was nearly proportionate across income groups. Based on this result, she concluded that that while medicare redistributes across income groups, this was largely the result of higher utilization of medicare services among lower-income groups as opposed to equity in financing. It should be borne in mind that health premiums – in effect, a regressive poll tax – still form part of the health financing mix in British Columbia. Since health premiums do not exist or have been integrated into existing income tax systems, this could mean that other provinces have relatively more progressive health financing than British Columbia. However, similar empirical analyses of health financing have not yet been conducted on the other provinces.

7.3 User experience and equity of access to health care

7.3.1 User experience

In response to growing levels of public dissatisfaction (see section 2.9 and Table 7.2) originally rooted in the public cost cutting of the early to mid-1990s, there has been a discernible trend towards reforms that will make the health system more responsive to patients. This movement, loosely termed patient-centred care, has become increasingly important in Canada as described in section 2.9.5. It is too early to determine the impact of these changes along with other provincial and territorial reforms aimed at making the system more responsive.

Table 7.2

Patient views on waiting times, access and health systems, Canada and selected OECD countries, 2010 (% of respondents in Commonwealth Fund survey)

	% of respondents					
Country	Wait for elective surgery (>4 months)	Wait for specialist appointment (>2 months)	Difficulty getting after-hours care without going to ED	Access to doctor or nurse when sick	Wait to see doctor or nurse when sick (>5 days)	Overall view that health system needs fundamental change or rebuilding
Australia	18	28	59	65	14	75
Canada	25	41	65	45	33	61
France	7	28	63	62	17	58
Sweden	22	31	68	57	25	53
United Kingdom	21	19	38	70	8	37
United States	7	9	63	57	19	68

Source: Schoen, Osborn & Squires (2010).

In the past decade, patient dissatisfaction has focused on the long waiting times for advanced diagnostics, specialist services and elective (non-urgent) surgery. Waiting times have also been an issue in some hospital emergency departments in urban centres. Finally, access to primary care – especially in those communities where there is a shortage of family physicians or where family physicians are refusing to take on new patients – has also fuelled patient dissatisfaction. These problems are reflected in a comparative study conducted by the Commonwealth Fund in 2010 (Schoen, Osborn & Squires, 2010).

Table 7.2 presents the results of the Commonwealth Fund's survey data for Canada and its five comparator countries. In terms of the patient experience with waiting times for elective surgery, specialist services and basic medical care access, Canada ranks behind Australia, France, Sweden, the United Kingdom and the United States. However, when it comes to the pressure on emergency rooms after regular hours due to the lack of 24/7 primary care, Canadians face roughly the same difficulty as patients in Australia, France, Sweden and the United States. In light of these poor results, it is not surprising that a majority of Canadians (61% in the sample) feel that the health system is in need of either major reform or rebuilding compared with the much larger percentage of Australians and Americans that have come to the same conclusion about their respective health systems.

7.3.2 Equity of access to health care

The introduction of universal medicare improved access to, and the benefits derived from, hospital and physician services (Enterline et al., 1973; van Doorslaer & Masseria, 2004; James et al., 2007). Despite this important public policy change in the 1950s and 1960s, inequities persist. Although these inequities are concentrated in non-medicare sectors where financing is largely private, they are also present in some services associated with medicare. Lower income Canadians tend to use acute inpatient services more than higher income Canadians but there is a pro-rich bias in terms of the use of specialist physician services, as well as day surgeries (Allin, 2008; McGrail, 2008).

While the evidence concerning primary care is mixed, one fine-grained study of British Columbia found that there was a higher use of primary care physicians among poorer Canadians (McGrail, 2008). One study found persistent inequities based on both education and income in the utilization of mental health services (Steele et al., 2007) – a troubling result given the increased incidence of mental illness in Canada. Other studies highlight the degree to which inequities exist in the use of non-medicare services, including dental care, rehabilitation, physiotherapy, occupational therapy and speech pathology (Hutchison, 2007; Grignon et al., 2010).

In Canada, the goal of achieving greater regional equity has also shaped health system financing. This "geographical" equity is pursued through two instruments: the first is equalization and the second is the Canada Health Transfer, two of the federal government's largest annual expenditures. First introduced when universal hospital insurance was established nationally, equalization payments from the federal government provide provincial governments that have shallower tax bases with the funding capacity to administer programmes such as medicare. By the early 1980s, equalization was considered such an important dimension of the federation that it was made part of the Canadian Constitution, and section 36(2) of the Constitution Act 1982 stipulates that the Government of Canada is required to make "equalization payments to ensure that provincial governments have sufficient revenues to provide reasonably comparable levels of public services at reasonably comparable levels of taxation".

The Canada Health Transfer provides both explicit and implicit regional redistribution. Through the Canada Health Transfer, revenues that are collected on a national basis are redistributed to the provinces, and those provinces with shallower tax bases benefit from the revenues collected in provinces with deeper pockets. There is also explicit equalization currently built into the Canada Health Transfer that assists less wealthy provinces. Under the Canada Health Transfer and its predecessor, the Canada Health and Social Transfer, the formula that calculated the share of each province involved a degree of equalization in which less wealthy provinces received slightly more per capita than wealthier provinces. After 2014, this element of equalization is to be terminated in favour of pure per capita payments. Nonetheless, as long as federal revenues fund some portion of provincial health care costs, there is some redistribution from wealthier parts of the country (where taxpayers pay more federal income and corporate taxes) to less wealthy parts of the country – an implicit form of revenue redistribution that would not exist if provinces alone raised revenues for their own health care expenditures.

7.4 Health outcomes, health service outcomes and quality of care

7.4.1 Population health and amenable mortality

Since the trends in health status have already been summarized in section 1.5, this section will focus on improvements in population health that can be attributed to the health system. It is extremely difficult to disentangle the contribution of the health system to health, through organized programmes, policies and interventions to prevent and treat illness and injury. In the face of these difficulties, successive researchers have refined an approach known as amenable mortality to isolate the impact of the health system from the other determinants of health.

Amenable mortality refers to death from selected diseases where death would not occur if those individuals had access to timely and effective health care. By isolating where death could be avoided and the condition in question treated (at least until a certain age), amenable mortality seeks to capture the extent to which the health system has, or has not, been effective at avoiding death (Nolte & McKee, 2004, 2008). This methodology is based on a host of mortality indicators that are then aggregated in a single amenable mortality scale.

Table 7.3

Amenable mortality rates and rank in Canada and selected OECD countries for last available year

	Last available year of data	Amenable mortality rate (age-standardized avoidable deaths per 100 000 population)	Rank among 31 OECD countries	Annual rate of change in amenable mortality from 1997 to last available year (%)
Australia	2004	68	7	-5.1
Canada	2004	74	11	-3.4
France	2006	59	1	-2.8
Sweden	2006	68	5	-3.3
United Kingdom	2007	86	19	-5.2
United States	2005	103	24	-1.7

Source: Gay et al. (2011).

Table 7.3 highlights the results of Canada and its comparators based on a larger study of 31 OECD countries in which age-standardized avoidable mortality ranged from a low of 59 to a high of 200 deaths per 100 000 population (Gay et al., 2011). While Canada's amenable mortality rate was at the low end, it did not rank as high as France (in first position), Sweden and Australia. On the other hand, Canada performed considerably better than the United Kingdom and the United States. In addition, the annual rate of decline in amenable mortality, although substantially slower than the rates in Australia and the United Kingdom, was modestly higher than the rates of decline in Sweden and France, and double the rate in the United States.

These results are consistent with a Canadian case study comparing the progress made (as measured by rates of decline in amenable mortality in the poorest neighbourhoods relative to the richest neighbourhoods) in 25 years following the introduction of universal medicare. While medicare has had an enormous impact on reducing the amenable mortality gap between poor and rich, this reduction in the disparity gap is due almost entirely to improving access to medical care as opposed to other types of health intervention. When examining amenable mortality in terms of public health interventions, there was little change over the same period, thus emphasizing the unrealized potential of public health policies, programmes and interventions (James et al., 2007).

This argument also applies to population health interventions – the so-called non-medical or social determinants of health. Despite the achievements made by Canadians in the early conceptualization on the importance of population health factors, it appears that the country's track record on the ground has been poor. Bryant et al. (2011) argued that ground has been ceded in the following five areas since the 1980s: (1) redistributive impact of tax and transfer policies; (2) family and child poverty; (3) housing policy; (4) early childhood education and care; and (5) urban and metropolitan health planning and policy.

7.4.2 Health service outcomes and quality of care

For years, the CIHI has been collecting and refining data in order to produce health service quality measures. Building an index of quality based on eight CIHI measures, Marchildon & Lockhart (2010) found that that there has been an overall trend towards quality improvement in Canada since the late 1990s (Fig. 7.1). While the OECD has recently launched a major quality indicators project, it is not yet possible to compare Canada with other OECD countries in terms of direct health service quality measures.

Fig. 7.1

Index and trend of eight quality indicators, 1999–2009

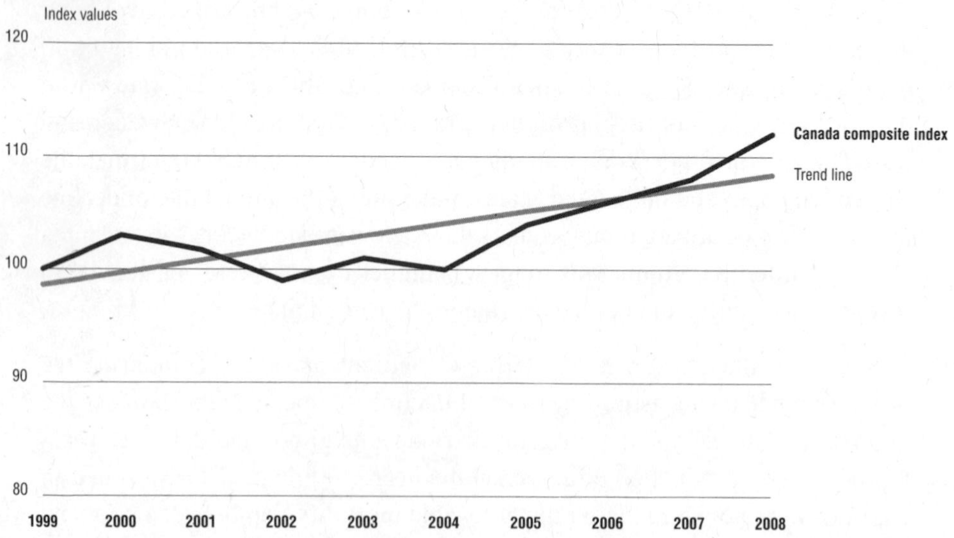

Source: Marchildon & Lockhart (2010).
Note: Although the eight CIHI indicators are focused on acute care, ambulatory sensitive conditions and hospital readmissions for particular conditions are used to determine the continuity of care beyond acute care and are therefore used as a broader measure of health system quality.

For the general public and health system decision-makers, waiting times have emerged as a major indicator of quality in Canada. As discussed in Chapter 6, first ministers identified five waiting time priority areas in the 10-Year Plan of 2004: cancer, heart, joint replacement, sight restoration and diagnostic imaging. They then asked their respective health ministers to produce a set of pan-Canadian benchmarks against which performance could be measured over time.

In 2005, health ministers produced six waiting time benchmarks for specific procedures in four of the five priority areas: (1) radiation therapy to treat cancer within four weeks; (2) cardiac bypass surgery within 2–26 weeks depending on the urgency of care; (3) surgery to remove cataracts within 16 weeks; (4) hip replacements within 26 weeks; (5) knee replacements within 26 weeks; and (6) surgical repair of hip fractures within 48 hours. While health ministers were unable to reach a consensus on pan-Canadian benchmarks for MRI and CT scans, some ministries of health have set their own waiting time thresholds for advanced diagnostics. Table 7.4 indicates that while most provinces have met or come close to meeting the benchmarks for cancer radiation therapy and cardiac bypass surgery, they still have some distance to go before they meet the waiting time benchmarks for joint replacement and sight restoration.

7.4.3 Equity of outcomes

As in other OECD countries, there is a robust relationship between socioeconomic status and health outcomes – the lower status the poorer are health outcomes. In Canada, there is also considerable evidence of a strong relationship between socioeconomic status and health care utilization – the lower education and income level of individuals, for example, the more likely they are to use more health care services (Mustard et al., 1997; Roos & Mustard, 1997; Curtis & MacMinn, 2008). The hard policy question is the extent to which existing and proposed health system interventions and services will improve health outcomes.

Table 7.4
Percentage of patients receiving care within pan-Canadian benchmarks, by province, 2011

	Radiation therapy for cancer (<4 weeks)	Cardiac bypass (<2–26 weeks)	Cataract removal (<16 weeks)	Hip replacement (<26 weeks)	Knee replacement (<26 weeks)	Hip fracture repair (<48 hours)
British Columbia	67	79	76	76	99	76
Alberta	98	95	59	80	70	81
Saskatchewan	99	100	58	75	62	84
Manitoba	100	97	71	59	52	85
Ontario	97	100	88	90	85	78
Quebec	99	–[a]	88	82	78	–[a]
New Brunswick	95	99	85	72	53	83
Nova Scotia	83	100	65	62	44	79
Prince Edward Island	96	–[b]	67	71	55	81
Newfoundland and Labrador	96	100	71	82	62	87
Canada	**97**	**99**	**82**	**82**	**75**	**79**

Source: CIHI (2012b). [a] Data provided in a form that was not comparable to other jurisdictions and therefore omitted;
[b] There are no cardiac bypass surgeons in Prince Edward Island and residents are sent to other provinces for this health service.

Some additional light has been thrown on this question by various scholars who have analysed the results of the Joint Canada–United States Survey of Health, 2002–2003. Both countries demonstrate a positive correlation between income and population health, but in the lowest income quintile, Canadians are healthier than Americans. Similarly, at lower levels of education, Canadians are healthier than Americans, a result attributed at least in part to the policy of universal medicare (Lasser, Himmelstein & Woolhandler, 2006; Eng & Feeny, 2007; McGrail et al., 2009).

Certain socioeconomic groups, particularly Canadian Aboriginal populations, have extremely low health status and health outcomes relative to the majority of the population. In part because of its fiduciary responsibilities for First Nations and Inuit, the federal government has funded and administered a large number of targeted population and public health programmes in an effort to narrow the gap in health disparities. In recent years, provincial and territorial governments have also initiated targeted policies and programmes. Despite these many efforts, a significant health disparity remains (Frohlick, Ross & Richmond, 2006; Loppie Reading & Wien, 2009).

In the 2006 census, immigrants made up nearly 20% of the Canadian population, and this percentage is forecast to be in excess of 25% by 2031. In contrast to Aboriginal peoples, immigrants in Canada tend, on average, to be healthier at least as measured by age-standardized mortality rates. This is known as the healthy immigrant effect, an effect that declines as their years in Canada increase (Ng, 2011). In terms of access to health care services, the lack of language proficiency (in either English or French depending on province of residence) is a barrier, especially for immigrant women (Pottie et al., 2008). While there is evidence that barriers other than language, such as lower income and sociocultural differences, also act as barriers in accessing health care services, there are fewer health access disparities between immigrants and non-immigrants in Canada compared with immigrants and non-immigrants in the United States (Asanin & Wilson, 2008; Siddiqi, Zuberi & Nguyen, 2009). The exceptions to the healthy immigrant effect are women from the United States and sub-Saharan Africa (Ng, 2011).

There are other important gender differences in terms of health outcomes and health service patterns in Canada. In particular, there is some evidence that women, particularly older women, are less likely than men to receive critical care that they need, and are more likely to die from critical illnesses (Fowler et al., 2007). In addition, older women are at increased risk of receiving inappropriate medications. These results cannot be generalized across all domains in part because gender-based analyses are not a routine part of health research, including clinical trials, despite the Canadian Institute of Health Research's policy supporting gender-based analysis. More importantly, without further gender-based analyses, it is extremely difficult to understand the underlying reasons for these gender-based differences in outcomes (Bierman, 2007).

In Canada, the majority of voluntary caregivers are women. In addition, they work at this task, on average, much more intensively than men (Brazil et al., 2009). Women also occupy the vast majority of the lower paid health worker positions in hospitals and long-term care homes and carry out the tasks of cleaning and caring for patients and residents. They also occupy most of the ancillary and support positions in health system (Armstrong, Armstrong & Scott-Dixon, 2006).

7.5 Health system efficiency

7.5.1 Allocative efficiency

Allocative efficiency stipulates that a health system distributes services in "accord with the value that individuals place on those goods and services" (Hurley, 2010, p.36). Where health goods and services are funded privately – as in roughly 30% of health spending in Canada – this will be done through the market as mediated or altered by PHI. In the case of publicly funded health services, allocative efficiency is more difficult to determine. Indeed, the economic notion of allocative efficiency may have little meaning as applied to public spending on health except in terms of whether governments have reached an appropriate balance in allocating funding among resource inputs (e.g. capital investment versus workforce inputs versus prescription drugs) and service sectors (e.g. public health versus primary care versus acute care versus long-term care).

Provincial and territorial health systems are funded through general tax revenues, thus offering governments considerable latitude in the allocation of expenditures among resource inputs and service sectors (see Chapter 3). Budgeting processes require that provincial government cabinets and their respective subcommittees – especially treasury board committees of cabinet – allocate among competing needs across a myriad of economic and social policy and programme demands. Since provincial governments ramped up health care spending after the years of restraint in the 1990s, it was argued by some that cabinet allocations to health care have crowded out other public needs (Boothe & Carson, 2003; MacKinnon, 2004). However, an empirical test of this hypothesis concluded that this was not the case (Landon et al., 2006).

Once ministries of health receive their budgets, they allocate among a number of health services and sectors based on the historic needs and demands of the sector as well as health policy and reform priorities as communicated by cabinet. In regionalized jurisdictions, the majority of ministry funding is distributed to RHAs based on a variety of methodologies, including population needs-based formulas, activity-based calculations, historically based budgeting and the government's immediate policy priorities. However, there have been few empirical comparisons of these different methodologies and their impact in terms of allocative efficiency.

7.5.2 Technical efficiency

Technical efficiency indicates the extent to which a health system draws on the minimum levels of inputs for a given output or, the maximum level of output based on a given set of inputs. To identify possible technical efficiencies, health system managers will ask whether it is possible to get more outputs with the same inputs, or whether it is possible to get the same output with fewer inputs (Hurley, 2010).

There have been few studies of the technical efficiency of health systems in Canada, in part because of the challenge posed by the large number of inputs as well as outputs in a complex health system whether it is a RHA or a provincial health system. However, there is increasing interest among OECD countries, including Canada, in conducting some "value for money" assessments (OECD, 2010a,b).

At least to some extent, the recent application of "lean production" methodologies in some provincial health systems and RHAs is an effort to achieve greater technical efficiency. First developed by the Japanese care manufacturer Toyota to achieve greater technical efficiency and higher quality in automobile production, lean techniques were first adapted to three hospitals in Ontario in 2005, followed by a RHA and a Catholic hospital in Saskatchewan one year later. The objective of these lean projects ranged from reducing surgical waiting times to improving patient safety (Fine et al., 2009). There has not yet been a systematic evaluation of these and subsequent lean initiatives in Canada, but one comparative study of its impact on 15 hospital emergency departments in three countries – Australia, Canada and the United States – found that there was a decrease in waiting times, total length of stay and the proportion of patients leaving emergency departments without being diagnosed or treated, as well as improvements in patient satisfaction (Holden, 2011).

7.6 Transparency and accountability

Health systems in Canada are more transparent today than in decades past due to a number of trends and movements. Canadians, whether in their various roles as citizen, taxpayer or patient, demand greater transparency of their governments and health care organizations than in the past. On the supply side, they now have access to information from a number of new provincial and intergovernmental organizations including the Health Council Canada, which provides accessible reports on the state of Canadian health care. In addition, a number of think tanks also provide reports on health system issues that are of concern and interest to Canadians.

Health Canada provides a yearly report to governments and the general public on the Canada Health Act, including any information concerning provincial governments that may be in breach of the Act and its five basic criteria of public administration, comprehensiveness, universality, portability and accessibility (Health Canada, 2011). However, concerns have been raised about what is actually included in the basket of universal health services under the Canada Health Act. In particular, private citizens have occasionally taken their provincial governments to court to have certain services added to the basket using arguments based on the Charter of Rights and Freedoms, and at least one scholar has argued that this is a useful mechanism for health care accountability, particularly given the paucity of other processes available to Canadian citizens (Jackman, 2010).

The Canada Health Act also stipulates that provincial and territorial governments should acknowledge the transfer funding they receive from the federal government, which is used to deliver public health care services to their respective residents. Demands for greater transparency in terms of federal transfers to provincial and territorial governments for health eventually led to the federal government splitting its omnibus block transfer into two in 2004 – the Canada Health Transfer dedicated to health, and the Canada Social Transfer (McIntosh, 2004). This came years after federal–provincial wrangling over what was the "real" value of the health portion of the block transfer, with the federal government continually exaggerating its value, and the provincial governments systematically underestimating its value (Marchildon, 2004).

Through their web sites, most provincial and territorial ministries of health provide extensive information on their services, including a comprehensive list of the provincial or territorial health care benefits and entitlements. With some notable exceptions, provincial and territorial governments have also been relatively transparent in terms of new health policy developments, in part because of their extensive and public use of commissions and ministerial advisory bodies during the past two decades. Inevitably, these processes have involved public consultations and hearings. The Royal Commission on the Future of Health Care in Canada, chaired by Roy Romanow, the former Premier of Saskatchewan, conducted the most extensive set of consultations with Canadians. Between 2001 and 2002, the Romanow Commission sponsored open public hearings, televised forums, expert workshops, regional forums, partnered dialogue sessions and a series of 12 one-day deliberative dialogue sessions involving a random selection of almost 500 Canadian citizens (Romanow, 2002; Maxwell et al., 2002; Maxwell, Rosell & Forest, 2003).

Beyond participating in parliamentary politics at the F/P/T levels of government, direct public involvement in health governance has been limited to more regional and local levels (Flood & Archibald, 2005). While there was a movement towards citizen election to RHA boards in the early days of regionalization, almost all RHA boards are now appointed by provincial governments (Abelson & Eyles, 2004; Chessie, 2009) (see section 2.9).

In terms of holding governments and other public actors to account for the management of health systems at the national, provincial, regional and local levels, Canadians have benefited from more public reporting on indicators and performance measures. The work of the CIHI since its establishment in 1994 has been critical in providing the infrastructure and comparative methodologies to allow this to occur (Morris & Zelmer, 2005). In addition, the HCC's mandate to provide health system information in an accessible form has also facilitated this type of public accountability. The council's recent release of a popular guide to health indicators reflects this mandate (HCC, 2011c).

8. Conclusions

In Canada, public and private coverage for health services is highly segmented by health sector. Universal, first-dollar coverage is restricted to medically necessary hospital and physician services. Other health goods and services, including prescription drugs, rehabilitative care and long-term care, are subject to targeted coverage or subsidies that cover some of the gaps left by PHI and OOP payments, but where private funds are the major source of financing, such as dental care, there are high levels of inequity in utilization and health outcomes.

Setting and achieving pan-Canadian standards and objectives in a highly decentralized federation requires considerable intergovernmental and intra-provincial collaboration. The last two decades have produced a dense network of intergovernmental agencies. While collaboration has succeeded in some areas (e.g. ensuring universal accessibility to hospital and physician services), it has been less effective in other areas (e.g. more effective use of IT). National standards are extremely difficult to achieve in sectors other than hospital and physician services. Historically, major shifts in policy direction may be easier to achieve in unitary states with centralized health systems, but decentralized systems may offer more opportunities for experimentation, as well as a rich environment for evaluating natural experiments. This is the potential offered by provincial health systems in Canada, a potential that could be more fully exploited in future years.

While there has been a discernible movement to greater patient empowerment in Canada in recent years, it remains relatively underdeveloped compared with similar movements in most other OECD countries. This is despite the fact that Canadians have a relatively poor view of at least some dimensions of their system, including timeliness and patient responsiveness. Such low satisfaction poses a challenge to Canadian Governments that have focused on improving the timeliness, quality and safety of health care. Recently, there have been improvements in quality outcomes as well as reductions in waiting times.

As for health expenditure, Canada is almost identical to other OECD countries in terms of its recent experience, although the precise sources of cost pressures may vary. One of the most important recent cost drivers is health sector inflation, due mainly to recent increases in physician and nurse remuneration, as well as payments to other health care workers (CIHI, 2011b). This has been accompanied by a major increase in the utilization of prescription drugs.

Overall, there has been a major reinvestment in public health care in Canada since the budget cutting of the early to mid-1990s. This has resulted in more doctors and nurses as well as an increase in the proportion of both relative to the general population. In addition, governments have invested heavily in capital infrastructure including medical equipment. In terms of imaging technologies such as CT and MRI scanners, Canada ranks average or higher than average among its OECD comparators. In a sense, Canadians have come full circle, from feast in the 1980s, to famine in the 1990s, and back to feast in the 2000s.

The results of setting health reform priorities through F/P/T agreements have been mixed to poor. The decision by the federal government not to participate in future first minister meetings is in part a judgement on the lack of success in the past as well as a political view that the federal government should not be involved in an area that is within the primary constitutional jurisdiction of the provinces. With most governments in Canada running budget deficits, the lack of discussion between the two orders of government reduces the possibility of reaching a pan-Canadian consensus on health priorities in the years to come. As a consequence, innovation is more likely to come from individual provinces and territories in a more constrained fiscal environment than the one that governments in Canada enjoyed during the past decade.

9. Appendices

9.1 References

Abelson J, Eyles J (2004). Public participation and citizen governance in the Canadian health system. In: Forest PG, Marchildon GP, McIntosh T, eds. *Changing health care in Canada*. Toronto, University of Toronto Press:279–311.

ACHDHR (2007). *A framework for collaborative health human resource planning*. Ottawa, Health Canada on behalf of the Advisory Committee on Health Delivery and Human Resources.

ACHDHR (2009). *How many are enough? Redefining self-sufficiency for the health workforce, a discussion paper*. Ottawa, Health Canada on behalf of the Advisory Committee on Health Delivery and Human Resources.

Adams D (2001). Canadian federalism and the development of national health goals and objectives. In: Adams D, ed. *Federalism, democracy and health policy in Canada*. Montreal, McGill-Queen's University Press:61–105.

Alberta Health and Wellness (2002). *A sustainable health system for Alberta: report of the MLA Task Force on Health Care Funding and Revenue Generation*. Edmonton, Alberta Health and Wellness.

Allin S (2008). Does equity in healthcare use vary across Canadian provinces. *Healthcare Policy*, 3(4):83–99.

Anis AH (2000). Pharmaceutical policies in Canada: another example of federal provincial discord. *Canadian Medical Association Journal*, 162(4):523–526.

Armstrong P, Armstrong H, Scott-Dixon K (2006). *Critical to care: women and ancillary work in health care*. Toronto, Women and Health Care Reform.

Asanin J, Wilson K (2008). "I spent nine years looking for a doctor": exploring access to health care among immigrants in Mississauga, Ontario, Canada. *Social Science & Medicine*, 66(6):1271–1283.

Auditor General of Canada (2009). *Report of the Auditor General of Canada to the House of Commons: Fall 2009*. Ottawa, Minister of Public Works and Government Services Canada.

Axelsson R, Marchildon GP, Repullo-Labrador JR (2007). Effects of decentralization on managerial dimensions of health systems. In: Saltman RB, Bankauskaite V, Vrangbæk K, eds. *Decentralization in health care*. New York: McGraw-Hill for European Observatory on Health Systems and Policies:141–166.

Babcock RH (2006). Blood on the factory floor: the workers' compensation movement in Canada and the United States. In: Blake RB, Keshen JA, eds. *Social fabric or patchwork quilt: the development of social policy in Canada*. Peterborough, ON: Broadview Press:45–58.

Badgley RF, Wolfe S (1967). *Doctor's strike: medical care and conflict in Saskatchewan.* Toronto: Macmillan of Canada.

Baker LC, Atlas SW, Afendulis CC (2008). Expanded use of imaging technology and the challenge of measuring value. *Health Affairs*, 27(6):1467–1478.

Ball GDC, McCargar LJ (2003). Childhood obesity in Canada: a review of prevalence estimates and risk factors for cardiovascular diseases and type 2 diabetes. *Canadian Journal of Applied Physiology,* 28(1):117–140.

Bates J, Lovato C, Buller-Taylor T (2008). "Mind the gap": seven key issues in aligning medical education and healthcare policy. *Healthcare Policy*, 4(2):46–58.

Battista RN, et al. (2009). Health technology assessment in Canada. *International Journal of Techology Assessment in Health Care*, 25 (suppl):53–60.

Bégin M (1988). *Medicare: Canada's right to health.* Ottawa, Optimum Publishing.

Berta W, Laporte A, Valdamanis V (2005). Observations on long-term care in Ontario, 1996–2002. *Canadian Journal of Aging*, 24(1):71–84.

Berta W, et al. (2006). A pan-Canadian perspective on institutional long-term care. *Health Policy*, 79(2–3):175–194.

Bierman AS (2007). Sex matters: gender disparities in quality and outcomes of care. *Canadian Medical Association Journal*, 177(12):1520–1521.

Boessenkool KJ (2010). *Fixing the fiscal imbalance: turning GST revenues over to the provinces in exchange for lower transfers*. Calgary, School of Public Policy.

Boothe P, Carson M (2003). *What happened to health-care reform?* Toronto, CD Howe Institute.

Boswell-Purdy J, et al. (2007). Population health impact of cancer in Canada, 2001. *Chronic Disease in Canada,* 28(1–2):42–55.

Boychuk T (1999). *The making and meaning of hospital policy in the United States and Canada*. Ann Arbor, University of Michigan Press.

Boychuk T (2009). After medicare: regionalization and Canadian health care reform. *Canadian Bulletin of Medical History*, 26(2):353–378.

Boyle S (2011). *Health systems in transition: United Kingdom (England)*. Copenhagen, WHO Regional Office for Europe on behalf of the European Observatory on Health Systems and Policies.

Braën A (2004). Health and the distribution of powers in Canada. In: McIntosh T, Forest PG, Marchildon GP, eds. *The governance of health care in Canada*. Toronto, University of Toronto Press:25–49.

Brazil K, et al. (2009). Gender differences among Canadian spousal caregivers at the end of life. *Health and Social Care in the Community*, 17(2):159–166.

Bryant T, et al. (2011). Canada: a land of missed opportunity for addressing the social determinants of health. *Health Policy*, 101(1):44–55.

Bullard MJ, et al. (2009). Tracking emergency department overcrowding in a tertiary care academic institution. *Healthcare Quarterly*, 12(3):99–106.

CADTH (2006). *Emergency department overcrowding in Canada: what are the issues and what can be done?* Ottawa, Canadian Agency for Drugs and Technologies in Health.

CADTH (2011). *Impact and change: 2009–2010 annual report.* Ottawa, Canadian Agency for Drugs and Technologies in Health.

Canada (1964). *Royal commission on health services,* Volume I. Ottawa, Queen's Printer.

Canada (2011). *Federal emergency response plan.* Ottawa, Government of Canada.

Canada Health Infoway (2003). *EHRS blueprint: an interoperable EHR framework.* Montreal, Canada Health Infoway.

Canada Health Infoway (2006). *EHRS blueprint: an interoperable EHR framework.* Montreal, Canada Health Infoway.

Canadian Council on Learning (2007). *Health Literacy in Canada: initial results from the International Adult Literacy and Skills Survey.* Ottawa, Canadian Council on Literacy.

Canadian Healthcare Association (2009). *Home care in Canada: from the margins to the mainstream.* Ottawa, Canadian Healthcare Association.

Canada Union Public Employees (2005). *Innovation exposes: an ongoing inventory of major privatization initiatives in Canada's health care system, 2004–2005.* Ottawa, Canadian Union of Public Employees.

Cancer Care Ontario (2010). *Ontario breast cancer screening program 20th anniversary report.* Toronto, Cancer Care Ontario.

Caulfield T (2004). Medical malpractice, the common law, and healthcare reform. In: Marchildon GP, McIntosh T, Forest PG, eds. *The fiscal sustainability of health care in Canada.* Toronto, University of Toronto Press:80–109.

Chafe R, Levinson W, Sullivan T (2009). Disclosing errors that affect multiple patients. *Canadian Medical Association Journal*, 180(11):1125–1127.

Chan B (2002a). *From perceived surplus to perceived shortage. What happened to Canada's physician workforce in the 1990s?* Ottawa, Canadian Institute for Health Information.

Chan B (2002b). The declining comprehensiveness of primary care. *Canadian Medical Association Journal*, 166(4):429–434.

Chan P, Kenny SR (2002). National consistency and provincial diversity in delivery of long-term care in Canada. *Journal of Aging and Social Policy,* 13(2–3):83–99.

Chessie K (2009). Health system regionalization in Canada's provincial and territorial health systems: do citizen governance boards represent, engage and empower? *International Journal of Health Services*, 39(4):705–724.

Chessie K (2010). The shifting discourse of "public participation": implications in changing models of health system regionalization. In: McIntosh T, Jeffery B, Muhajarine N, eds. *Redistributing health: new directions in population health research in Canada.* Regina, CPRC Press:74–92.

Chevreul K, et al. (2010). *Health Systems in Transition: France.* Copenhagen, WHO Regional Office for Europe on behalf of the European Observatory on Health Systems and Policies.

Canadian Hospice Palliative Care Association (2002). *Model to guide hospice palliative care: based on national principles and norms of practice.* Ottawa, Canadian Hospice Palliative Care Association.

CICS (2003). *2003 First ministers' accord on health care renewal.* Ottawa, Canadian Intergovernmental Conference Secretariat (5 February 2003).

CICS (2004). *A 10-Year plan to strengthen health care.* Ottawa, Canadian Intergovernmental Conference Secretariat (16 September 2004).

CIHI (2008a). *Inpatient rehabilitation in Canada, 2006–2007.* Ottawa, Canadian Institute for Health Information.

CIHI (2008b). *Medical imaging in Canada 2007.* Ottawa, Canadian Institute for Health Information.

CIHI (2010a). *Highlights of 2008–2009 inpatient hospitalizations and emergency department visits.* Ottawa, Canadian Institute for Health Information.

CIHI (2010b). *National health expenditure trends, 1975–2010.* Ottawa, Canadian Institute for Health Information.

CIHI (2010c). *National physician database, 2008–2009.* Ottawa, Canadian Institute for Health Information.

CIHI (2010d). *Regulated nurses: Canadian trends, 2005 to 2009.* Ottawa, Canadian Institute for Health Information.

CIHI (2010e). *Supply, distribution and migration of Canadian physicians.* Ottawa, Canadian Institute for Health Information.

CIHI (2011a). *Canada's health care providers, 2000 to 2009: a reference guide.* Ottawa, Canadian Institute for Health Information.

CIHI (2011b). *Health care cost drivers: the facts.* Ottawa, Canadian Institute for Health Information.

CIHI (2011c). *Health indicators 2011.* Ottawa, Canadian Institute for Health Information.

CIHI (2011d). *Highlights of the 2009–2010 inpatient hospital and emergency department visits.* Ottawa, Canadian Institute for Health Information.

CIHI (2011e). *National health expenditure trends, 1975–2011.* Ottawa, Canadian Institute for Health Information.

CIHI (2011f). *National physician database, 2009–2010: data release.* Ottawa, Canadian Institute for Health Information.

CIHI (2012a). *National survey of selected medical imaging equipment.* Ottawa, Canadian Institute for Health Information (http://www.cihi.ca/cihi-ext-portal/internet/en/tabbedcontent/types+of+care/specialized+services/medical+imaging/cihi010642, accessed 11 March 2012).

CIHI (2012b). *Wait times in Canada: a summary, 2012.* Ottawa, Canadian Institute for Health Information.

Cinnamon B (2009). *Results from the Functional Foods and Natural Health Products Survey, 2007.* Ottawa, Statistics Canada (Business Special Survey and Technology Statistics Division working paper).

Clarke JN (2004). *Health, illness, and medicine in Canada,* 4th edn. Toronto, Oxford University Press.

Clatney L, MacDonald H, Shah SM (2008). Mental health care in the primary setting: family physicians' perspectives. *Canadian Family Physician*, 54(6):884–889.

College of Nurses of Ontario (2004). *Registered nurses in the extended class.* Toronto, College of Nurses of Ontario.

Cousin M (2009). Health care and human rights after Auton and Chaoulli. *McGill Law Journal*, 54(4):717–738.

Coyte PC, Landon S (1990). Cost-sharing and block-funding in a federal system: a demand systems approach. *Canada Journal of Economics*, 23(4):817–838.

CPSI (2008). *Canadian disclosure guidelines*. Edmonton, Canadian Patient Safety Institute.

CPSI (2011). *Canadian disclosure guidelines: being open with patients and families*. Edmonton, Canadian Patient Safety Institute.

Crosato KE, Leipert B (2006). Rural women caregivers in Canada. *Rural and Remote Health*, 6(2): 52.

Curtis LJ, MacMinn WJ (2008). Health care utilization in Canada: twenty-five years of evidence. *Canadian Public Policy*, 34(1):65–87.

Dagnone T (2009). *For patients' sake: Patient First Review Commissioner's report to the Saskatchewan Minister of Health*. Regina, Saskatchewan Ministry of Health.

Daw JR, Morgan SG (2012). Stitching the gaps in the Canadian public drug coverage patchwork: a review of provincial pharmacare policy changes from 2000 to 2010. *Health Policy*, 104(1): 19–26.

Deber RB (2004). Delivering health care: public, not-for-profit, or private? In: Marchildon GP, McIntosh T, Forest PG, eds. *The fiscal sustainability of health care in Canada*. Toronto, University of Toronto Press:233–296.

De Wals P (2011). Optimizing the acceptability, effectiveness and cost of immunization programs: the Quebec experience. *Expert Review of Vaccines*, 10(1):55–62.

Denis JL (2004). Governance and management of change in Canada's health system. In: Forest PG, Marchildon GP, McIntosh T, eds. *Changing health care in Canada*. Toronto, University of Toronto Press:82–114.

Donaldson C (2010). Fire, aim… ready? Alberta's big bank approach to healthcare disintegration. *Healthcare Policy*, 6(1):22–31.

Duckett S (2010). Second wave reform in Alberta. *Healthcare Management Forum*, 25(4):156–158.

Dumont JC, et al. (2008). *International mobility of health professionals and health workforce management in Canada: myths and realities*. Paris, Organisation for Economic Co-operation and Development and World Health Organization.

Dumont S, et al. (2009). Costs associated with resource utilization during the palliative phase of care: a palliative perspective. *Palliative Medicine*, 23(8):708–717.

Dyck E (2011). Dismantling the asylum and charting new pathways into the community: mental health care in 20th century Canada. *Histoire Sociale/Social History*, 44(2):181–196.

Elections Canada (2008). Official voting results: fortieth general election 2008. Ottawa, Elections Canada (http://www.elections.ca/scripts/OVR2008/default.html, accessed 21 April 2011).

Elections Canada (2011). 2011 General election: preliminary results. Ottawa, Elections Canada (http://enr.elections.ca/National_e.aspx, accessed 22 May 2011).

Eng K, Feeny D (2007). Comparing the health of low income and less well-educated groups in the United States and Canada. *Population Health Metrics* 5:10 (online at: (http://www.pophealthmetrics.com/content/5/1/10, accessed 25 September 2012).

Enterline PE, et al. (1973). The distribution of medical services before and after "free" medical care: the Quebec experience. *New England Journal of Medicine*, 289(22):1174–1178.

Evans RG, McGrail KM (2008). Richard III, Barer-Stoddart and the daughter of time. *Healthcare Policy*, 3(3):18–28.

Expert Panel on Equalization and Territorial Formula Financing (2006). *Achieving a national purpose: putting equalization back on track*. Ottawa, Department of Finance Canada.

Fafard P (2012). Intergovernmental accountability and health care: reflections on the recent Canadian experience. In: Graefe P, Simmons JM, White LA, eds. *Overpromising and underperforming? Understanding and evaluating new intergovernmental accountability regimes*. Toronto, University of Toronto Press: 31–55.

Fast J, et al. (2004). Characteristics of family/friend care networks of frail seniors. *Canadian Journal of Aging*, 23(1):5–19.

Fenna A (2010). *Benchmarking in federal systems*. Ottawa, Forum of the Federations.

Fine BA, et al. (2009). Leading lean: a Canadian healthcare leader's guide. *Healthcare Quarterly*, 12(3):32–41.

Flagler J, Dong W (2010). The uncompassionate elements of the Compassionate Care Benefits Program: a critical analysis. *Global Health Promotion*, 17(1):50–59.

Flegel KM, Hébert PC, MacDonald N (2008). Is it time for another medical curriculum revolution? *Canadian Medical Associatiom Journal*, 178(1):11.

Flood CM (2007). Chaoulli's legacy for the future of Canadian health care policy. In: Campbell B, Marchildon GP, eds. The governance of health care in Canada. Toronto: James Lorimer:256–191.

Flood CM (2010). The evidentiary burden for overturning government's choice of regulatory instrument: the case of direct-to-consumer advertising of prescription drugs. *University of Toronto Law Journal*, 60(2):397–424.

Flood CM, Archibald T (2001). The illegality of private health care in Canada. *Canadian Medical Association Journal*, 164(6):825–830.

Flood CM, Archibald T (2005). *Hamstrung and hogtied: cascading constraints on citizen governance in medicare*. Ottawa, Canadian Policy Research Networks.

Flood CM, Choudhry S (2004). Strengthening the foundations: modernizing the Canada Health Act. In: McIntosh T, Forest PG, Marchildon GP, eds. *The governance of health care in Canada*. Toronto: University of Toronto Press:346–387.

Flood, CM, Roach K, Sossin L (2005). *Access to care, access to justice: the legal debate over private health insurance in Canada*. Toronto: University of Toronto Press.

Flood CM, Stabile M, Tuohy C (2006). What is in and out of medicare? Who decides? In: Flood CM, ed. *Just medicare: What's in, what's out, how we decide*. Toronto, University of Toronto Press.

Fowler RA, et al. (2007). Sex and age-based differences in the delivery and outcomes of critical care. *Canadian Medical Assocation Journal*, 177(12):1513–1519.

Frohlick KL, Ross N, Richmond C (2006). Health disparities in Canada today: some evidence and a theoretical framework. *Health Policy*, 79(2–3):132–143.

Gay JG, et al. (2011). *Mortality amenable to health care in 31 OECD countries*. Paris, Organisation for Economic Co-operation and Development.

Gechert S (2010). Supplementary private health insurance in selected countries: lessons for EU governments. *CESifo Economic Studies*, 56(3):444–464.

Gerdtham UG, Jönsson B (2000). International comparisons of health expenditure: theory, data and econometric analysis. In: Culyer AJ, Newhouse JP, eds. *Handbook of Health Economics,* Volume 1. Amsterdam, Elsevier:1–45.

Giacomini M, Miller F, Browman G (2003). Confronting the "grey zones" of technology assessment: evaluating genetic testing services for public insurance coverage in Canada. *International Journal of Technology Assessment in Health Care*, 19(2):301–315.

Glazier RH, et al. (2009). Capitation and enhanced fee-for-service models for primary care reform: a population-based evaluation. *Canadian Medical Association Journal*, 180(11):E72–E81.

Gilmour J, Kelner M, Wellman B (2002). Opening the door to complementary and alternative medicine: self-regulation in Ontario. Law & Policy, 24(2):149–174.

Glauser W (2011). Private clinics continue explosive growth. *Canadian Medical Association Journal*, 183(8):E437–E438.

Golding L (2005). *Wait times: legal issues – patient rights*. Toronto, Fasken Martineau DuMoullin LLP, National Health Law Group.

Government of Canada (2002). *A national assessment of emergency planning in Canada's general hospitals*. Ottawa, Government of Canada, Office of Critical Infrastructure Protection and Emergency Preparedness.

Greschner D (2004). How will the Charter of Rights and Freedoms and evolving jurisprudence affect health care costs? In: McIntosh T, Forest PG, Marchildon GP, eds. *The governance of health care in Canada*. Toronto, University of Toronto Press:83–124.

Grignon M, Paris V, Polton D (2004). The influence of physician-payment methods on the efficiency of the health care system. In: Forest PG, Marchildon GP, McIntosh T, eds. *Changing health care in Canada*. Toronto, University of Toronto Press:207–240.

Grignon M, et al. (2010). Inequity in a market-based health system: evidence from Canada's dental sector. *Health Policy*, 98(1):81–90.

Grishaber-Otto J, Sinclair S (2004). *Bad medicine: trade treaties, privatization and health care reform in Canada*. Ottawa, Canadian Centre for Policy Alternatives.

Grootendorst P, Hollis A (2011). *Managing pharmaceutical expenditures: overview and options for Canada*. Ottawa, Canadian Health Services Research Foundation.

Grzybowski S, Allen EA (1999). Tuberculosis: 2. History of the disease in Canada. *Canadian Medical Association Journal*, 160(7):1025–1028.

Hailey DM (2007). Health technology assessment in Canada: diversity and evolution. *Medical Journal of Australia*, 187:286–288.

Hall, EM (1980). *Canada's national-provincial health program for the 1980s*. Ottawa, National Health and Welfare, 1980.

HCC (2009). *A status report on the National Pharmaceuticals Strategy: a prescription unfilled*. Toronto, Health Council of Canada.

HCC (2010a). *Decisions, decisions: family doctors as gatekeepers to prescription drugs and diagnostic imaging in Canada*. Toronto, Health Council of Canada.

HCC (2010b). *Stepping it up: moving the focus from health care in Canada to a healthier Canada – Appendix A: selected provincial, territorial and federal horizontal initiatives and whole-of-government approaches to improve population health and reduce inequalities*. Toronto, Health Council of Canada.

HCC (2011a). *A citizen's guide to health indicators: a reference guide for Canadians*. Toronto, Health Council of Canada.

HCC (2011b). *How engaged are Canadians in their primary health care? Results from the 2010 Commonwealth Fund International Health Policy Survey*. Toronto, Health Council of Canada.

Health Canada (2002). *Federal nuclear emergency plan, part 1: master plan*. Ottawa, Health Canada.

Health Canada (2003). *Learning from SARS: renewal of public health*. Ottawa, Health Canada.

Health Canada (2007). *Medical devices program strategic plan, 2007–2012: building for the future*. Ottawa, Health Canada.

Health Canada (2010). *Report on the findings of the oral health component of the Canadian Health Measures Survey, 2007–2009*. Ottawa, Health Canada.

Health Canada (2011). *Canada Health Act: annual report, 2009–2010*. Ottawa, Health Canada.

Health Charities Council of Canada (2001). *Increasing wellness in Canadians: the role of health charities*. Ottawa, Health Charities Council of Canada.

Health and Welfare Canada (1974). *A new perspective on the health of Canadians: the Lalonde report*. Ottawa, Health and Welfare Canada.

Healy J, McKee J (2002). The role and function of hospitals. In: McKee M, Healy J, eds. *Hospitals in a changing Europe*. Buckingham, UK, Open University Press:59–80.

Hillman BJ, Goldsmith JC (2010). The uncritical use of high-tech medical imaging. *New England Journal of Medicine*, 363(1):4–6.

Hirdes J (2002). Long-term care funding in Canada. *Journal of Aging and Social Policy*, 13(2–3):69–81.

Holden RJ (2011). Lean thinking in emergency departments: a critical review. *Annals of Emergency Medicine*, 57(3):265–278.

Hollander MJ, et al. (2009). Increasing value for money in the Canadian healthcare system: new findings and the case for integrated care for seniors. *Healthcare Quarterly*, 12(1):38–47.

Hollander MJ, Guiping L, Chappell NL (2009). Who cares and how much? The imputed economic contribution to the Canadian healthcare system of middle-aged and older unpaid caregivers providing care to the elderly. *Healthcare Quarterly*, 12(9):42–49.

Houston CS (2002). *Steps on the road to medicare: why Saskatchewan led the way*. Montreal, McGill-Queen's University Press.

HPRAC (2006). *Regulation of health professions in Ontario: new directions*. Toronto, Health Professions Regulatory Advisory Council.

HPRAC (2008). *An interim report to the Minister of Health and Long-Term Care on the mechanisms to facilitate and support interprofessional collaboration among health colleges and regulated health professions*. Toronto, Health Professions Regulatory Advisory Council.

Hu J, et al. (2006). Trends in mortality from ischemic heart disease in Canada, 1986–2000. *Chronic Diseases in Canada*, 27(2):85–91.

Hurley J (2010). *Health economics*. Toronto, McGraw-Hill Ryerson.

Hurley J, Guindon GE (2008). *Private health insurance in Canada*. Hamilton, McMaster University, Centre for Health Economics and Policy Analysis working paper.

Hurley J, Guindon GE (2011). *Private health insurance in Canada*. Hamilton, McMaster University, Centre for Health Economics and Policy Analysis updated version of 2008 the working paper, provided by author.

Hurley J, et al. (2008). Parallel lines do intersect: interactions between the workers' compensation and provincial publicly financed healthcare systems in Canada. *Healthcare Policy*, 3(4):100–112.

Hutchison B (2007). Disparaties in healthcare access and use: yackety-yack, yackety-yack. *Healthcare Policy*, 3(2):10–12.

Hutchison B, Abelson J, Lavis J (2001). Primary care in Canada: so much innovation, so little change. *Health Affairs*, 20(3):116–131.

Hutchison B, et al. (2011). Primary health care in Canada: systems in motion. *Milbank Quarterly*, 89(2):256–288.

ICES (2012). *Comparison of primary care models in Ontario by demographics, case mix and emergency department use, 2008/09 to 2009/10.* Toronto, Institute for Clinical Evaluative Sciences.

Ito D (2011). Oral health for all Ontarians: why not a future reality? In: Yalnizyan A, Aslanyan G, eds. *Putting our money where our month is: the future of dental care in Canada.* Ottawa, Canadian Centre for Policy Alternatives:18–19.

ITU (2011). *Measuring the information society, 2011.* Geneva, International Telecommunication Union.

Jackman M (2004). Section 7 of the Charter and health-care spending. In: Marchildon GP, McIntosh T, Forest PG, eds. *The fiscal sustainability of health care in Canada.* Toronto, University of Toronto Press:110–136.

Jackman M (2010). Charter review as a health care accountability mechanism in Canada. *Health Law Journal*, 18:1–29.

James PD, et al. (2007). Avoidable mortality by neighbourhood income in Canada: 25 years after the establishment of universal health insurance. *Journal of Epidemiology and Community Health*, 61(4): 287–296.

Jha AK, et al. (2008). The use of health information technology in seven nations. *International Journal of Medical Informatics*, 77(12):848–854.

Johnson JR (2004a). International trade agreements and Canadian health care. In: Marchildon GP, McIntosh T, Forest PG, eds. *The fiscal sustainability of health care in Canada.* Toronto, University of Toronto Press:369–402.

Johnson AW (2004b). *Dream no little dreams: a biography of the Douglas Government of Saskatchewan, 1944–1961.* Toronto: University of Toronto Press.

Jonas WB, Levin JS, eds. (1999). *Essentials of complementary and alternative medicine.* Philadelphia, Lippincott, Williams & Wilkins.

Kapur A (2003). Global solidarity against globalized tobacco: the world's first modern health treaty. *Canadian Medical Association Journal*, 168(10):1263–1264.

Katzmarzyk PT, Janssen I (2004). The economic costs associated with physical inactivity and obesity in Canada: an update. *Canadian Journal of Applied Physiology,* 29(1):90–115.

Katzmarzyk PT, Mason C (2006). Prevalence of class I, II and III obesity in Canada. *Canadian Medical Association Journal*, 174(2):156–157.

Kelner M, et al. (2004). Responses of established healthcare to the professions of CAM in Ontario. *Social Science & Medicine*, 59(5):915–930.

Kickbusch I (2003). The contribution of the World Health Organization to the new public health and health promotion. *American Journal of Public Health*, 93(3):383–388.

Lahey W, Currie R (2005). Regulatory and medico-legal barriers to interprofessional practice. *Journal of Interprofessional Care*, 19(suppl 1):197–223.

Lampard R (2009). The Hoadley Commission (1932–34) and health insurance in Alberta. *Canadian Bulletin of Medical History*, 26(2):429–452.

Landon S, et al. (2006). Does health-care spending crowd out other provincial government expenditures? *Canadian Public Policy*, 32(2):121–141.

Landry MD, et al. (2008). Shifting sands: assessing the balance between public, private not-for-profit and private-for-profit physiotherapy delivery in Ontario, Canada. *Physiotherapy Research International*, 13(3):189–199.

Landry MD, Raman S, Al-Hamdan E (2010). Accessing timely rehabilitation services for a global aging society? Exploring the realities within Canada's universal health care system. *Current Aging Science*, 3(2):143–4150.

Lasser KE, Himmelstein DU, Woolhandler S (2006). Access to care. Health status and health disparities in the United States and Canada: results from a cross-national population-based survey. *American Journal of Public Health*, 96(7):1300–1307.

Lavoie JG (2004). Governed by contracts: the development of indigenous primary health services in Canada, Australia and New Zealand. *Journal of Aboriginal Health,* 1(1):6–24.

Lawrence H, et al. (2009). Oral health inequaties between young Aboriginal and non-Aboriginal children living in Ontario, Canada. *Community Dentistry and Oral Epidemiology*, 37(6):495–508.

Lawson G, Noseworthy AF (2009). Newfoundland's cottage hospital system. *Canadian Bulletin of Medical History*, 26(2):477–498.

Lazar H, St-Hilaire F (2004). *Money, politics and health care: reconstructing the federal–provincial partnership*. Montreal, Institute for Research on Public Policy.

Leake JL, Birch S (2008). Public policy and the market for dental services. *Community Dentistry and Oral Epidemiology*, 36(4):287–295.

Lee DS, et al. (2009). Trends in risk factors of cardiovascular disease in Canada: temporal, socio-demographic and geographic factors. *Canadian Medical Association Journal,* 181(3–4):E55–E66.

Leeb K, Morris K, Kasman N (2005). Dying of cancer in Canada's acute care facilities. *Healthcare Quarterly*, 8(3):26–28.

Leeson H (2004). Constitutional jurisdiction over health and health care services in Canada. In: McIntosh T, Forest PG, Marchildon GP, eds. *The governance of health care in Canada*. Toronto, University of Toronto Press:50–82.

Léger PT (2011). *Physician payment mechanisms: an overview of policy options for Canada.* Ottawa, Canadian Health Services Research Foundation.

Lemchuk-Favel L, Jock JG (2004). Aboriginal health systems in Canada: nine case studies. *Journal of Aboriginal Health*, 1(1):6–24.

Lett W (2008). Private health clinics remain unregulated in most of Canada. *Canadian Medical Association Journal*, 178(8):986–987.

Levinson W, Gallagher TH (2007). Disclosing medical errors to patients: a status report in 2007. *Canadian Medical Association Journal*, 177(3):265–267.

Lewis S, Kouri D (2004). Regionalization: making sense of the Canadian experience. *Healthcare Papers*, 5(1):12–31.

Loppie Reading C, Wien F (2009). *Health inequalities and social determinants of Aboriginal Peoples health*. Prince George, National Collaborating Centre on Aboriginal Health.

Lozeau D (1999). Des rituels and des hommes: la gestion de la qualité en milieu hospitalier au Québec. *Canadian Public Administration*, 42(4):542–565.

MacDougall H (2009). Into thin air: making national health policy, 1939–45. *Canadian Bulletin of Medical History*, 26(2):283–313.

Mackenzie H (2004). *Financing Canada's hospitals: public alternatives to P3s*. Toronto, Hugh Mackenzie and Associates.

MacKinnon J (2004). The arithmetic of health care. *Canadian Medical Association Journal*, 171(6):603–604.

MacKinnon NJ, Ip I (2009). The national pharmaceuticals strategy: rest in peace, revive or renew? *Canadian Medical Association Journal*, 180(8):801–803.

Maddelena V (2006). Governance, public participation and accountability: to whom are regional health authorities accountable? *Healthcare Management Forum*, 19(3):30–35.

Makomaski IEM, Kaiserman MJ (2004). Mortality attributable to tobacco use in Canada and its regions, 1998. *Canada Journal of Public Health,* 95(1):38–44.

Marchildon GP (2004). *Three choices for the future of medicare*. Ottawa, Caledon Institute of Social Policy.

Marchildon GP (2005). *Health systems in transition: Canada*. Copenhagen, WHO Regional Office for Europe on behalf of the European Observatory on Health Systems and Policies.

Marchildon GP (2006). Regionalization and health services restructuring in Saskatchewan. In: Beach CM et al. *Health services restructuring in Canada: New evidence and new directions*, Montreal, McGill-Queen's University Press:33–57.

Marchildon GP (2007). Federal Pharmacare: prescription for an ailing federation? In: Campbell B, Marchildon GP, eds. *Medicare: facts, myths, problems and promise*. Toronto, Lorimer:268–284.

Marchildon GP (2008). Health security in Canada: policy complexity and overlap. *Social Theory & Health*, 6(1):74–90.

Marchildon GP (2009). The policy history of Canadian medicare. *Canadian Bulletin of Medical History,* 26(20):247–260.

Marchildon GP (2010). Health care. In: Courtney JC, Smith DE, eds. *The Oxford handbook of Canadian politics*. New York, Oxford University Press:434–450.

Marchildon GP (2011). Access to basic dental care in Canada and the heavy hand of history. In: Yalnizyan A, Aslanyan G, eds. *Putting our money where our mouth is: the future of dental care in Canada*. Ottawa, Canadian Centre for Policy Alternatives:20–22.

Marchildon GP, Chatwoods (2012). Northern Canada. *Circumpolar Health Supplements*, 2012(9):41–51.

Marchildon GP, Lockhart W (2010). Common trends in public stewardship of health care. In: Rosen B, Israeli A, Shortell S, eds. *Improving health and healthcare. Who is responsible? Who is accountable?* Jerusalem, Israeli National Institute for Health Policy Research on behalf of the Fourth International Jerusalem Conference:62–75.

Marchildon GP, O'Byrne NC (2009). From Bennettcare to medicare: the morphing of medical care insurance in British Columbia. *Canadian Bulletin of Medical History*, 26(2):453–475.

Marchildon GP, Schrijvers K (2011). Physician resistance and the forging of public health care: a comparative analysis of the doctors' strikes in Canada and Belgium in the 1960s. *Medical History*, 55(2):203–222.

Martens PJ, et al. (2002). *The health and health care use of registered First Nations people living in Manitoba: a population-based study*. Winnipeg, Manitoba Centre for Health Policy.

Maxwell J, et al. (2002). *Citizens' dialogue on the future of health care in Canada: report prepared for the Commission on the Future of Health Care in Canada*. Ottawa, Canadian Policy Research Networks.

Maxwell J, Rosell S, Forest PG (2003). Giving citizens a voice in healthcare policy in Canada. *BMJ*, 326(7397):1031–1033.

McDonnell TE, McDonnell DE (2005). Policy forum: taxing for health care: the Ontario model, 2004. *Canadian Tax Journal*, 53(1):107–134.

McGrail K (2007). medicare financing and redistribution in British Columbia, 1992 and 2002. *Health Policy*, 2(4):123–137.

McGrail K (2008). Income-related inequities: cross-sectional analyses of the use of medicare services in British Columbia in 1992 and 2002. *Open Medicine*, 2(4):e3–e10.

McGrail KM, et al. (2007). For-profit versus not-for-profit delivery of long-term care. *Canadian Medical Association Journal*, 176(1):57–58.

McGrail KM, et al. (2009). Income-related health inequities in Canada and the United States: a decomposition analysis. *American Journal of Public Health*, 99(10):1856–1863.

McIntosh T (2004). Intergovernmental relations, social policy and federal transfers after Romanow. *Canadian Public Administration*, 47(1):27–51.

McIntosh T, Ducie M (2009). Private health facilities in Saskatchewan: marginalizing through legalization. *Canadian Political Science Review*, 3(4):47–62.

McIntosh T, Torgerson R, Klassen N (2007). *The ethical recruitment of internationally educated health professionals: lessons from abroad and options for Canada*. Ottawa, Canadian Policy Research Networks.

McIntosh T, et al. (2010). Population health and health system reform: needs-based funding for health services in five provinces. *Canadian Political Science Review*, 4(1):42–61.

McKillop I (2004). Financial rules as a catalyst for change in the Canadian health care system. In: Forest PG, Marchildon GP, McIntosh T, eds. *Changing health care in Canada*. Toronto, University of Toronto Press.

McLeod L, et al. (2011). Financial burden of household out-of-picket expenditures for prescription drugs: cross-sectional analysis based on national survey data. *Open Medicine*, 5(1):e1–e9.

McMahon M, Morgan S, Mitton C (2006). The Common Drug Review: a NICE start for Canada? *Health Policy*, 77(3):339–351.

Menon D, Stafinski T (2009). Health technology assessment in Canada: 20 years strong? *Value in Health*, 12(suppl 2):S14–S19.

Menon D, Stafinski T, Stuart G (2005). Access to drugs for cancer: does where you live matter? *Canadian Journal of Public Health*, 96(6):454–458.

Mhatre SL, Deber RB (1992). From equal access to health care to equitable access to health: a review of Canadian provincial health commissions and reports. *International Journal of Health Services*, 22(4):645–668.

MHCC (2009). *Toward recovery and well-being: a framework for a mental health strategy for Canada*. Calgary, Mental Health Commission of Canada.

MHCC (2012). *Changing directions, changing lives: the mental health strategy for Canada*. Calgary, Mental Health Commission of Canada.

Middleton C, Veenhof B, Leith J (2010). *Intensity of internet use in Canada: understanding different types of users*. Ottawa, Statistics Canada, Business Special Surveys and Technical Statistics Division working paper.

Mills EJ, et al. (2011). The financial cost of doctors emigrating from sub-Saharan Africa: human capital analysis. *BMJ,* 343:d7031.

Minore B, Katt M (2007). *Aboriginal health care in northern Ontario: impacts of self-determination and culture.* Montreal, Institute of Research on Public Policy.

Mintzes B, et al. (2002). Influence of direct to consumer advertising and patients' requests on prescribing decisions: two site cross sectional survey. *BMJ,* 324:278–279.

Mohr J (2000). American medical malpractice litigation in historical perspective. *JAMA,* 283(13):1731–1737.

Morgan S, Hurley J (2004). Technological change as a cost-driver in health care. In: Marchildon GP, McIntosh T, Forest PG, eds. *The fiscal sustainability of health care in Canada.* Toronto, University of Toronto Press:27–50.

Morris K, Zelmer J (2005). *Public reporting on performance measures in health care.* Ottawa, Canadian Policy Research Networks.

Mulvale G, Abelson J, Goering P (2007). Mental health service delivery in Ontario, Canada: how do policy legacies shape prospects for reform. *Health Economics, Policy and Law,* 2(4):363–389.

Mustard CA, et al. (1997). Age-specific education and income gradients in morbidity and mortality in a Canadian province. *Social Science & Medicine,* 45(3):383–397.

NACI (2006). *The Canadian immunization guide, 7th eds.* Ottawa, Public Health Agency of Canada on behalf of the National Advisory Committee on Immunization.

Nahas R, Balla A (2011). Complementary and alternative medicine for prevention and treatment of the common cold. *Canadian Family Physician,* 57(1):31–36.

National Steering Committee on Patient Safety (2002). *Building a safer system: a national integrated strategy for improving patient safety in Canadian health care.* Edmonton, Canadian Patient Safety Institute.

Naylor CD (1986). *Private practice, public payment: Canadian medicine and the politics of health insurance, 1911–1966.* Montreal, McGill-Queen's University Press.

Ng E (2011). The healthy immigrant effect and mortality rates. *Statistics Canada Health Reports,* 22(4):1–5.

Ng E, Omariba DW (2010). *Health literacy and immigrants in Canada: determinants and effects on health outcomes.* Ottawa, Canadian Council on Learning.

Nicklin W (2011). *The value and impact of health care accreditation: a literature review.* Ottawa, Accreditation Canada.

Nolte E, McKee M (2004). *Does health care save lives? Avoidable mortality revisited.* London, Nuffield Trust.

Nolte E, McKee M (2008). Measuring the health of nations: updating an earlier analysis. *Health Affairs,* 27(1):58–71.

OECD (2008). *Mental health in OECD countries: policy brief.* Paris, Organisation for Economic Co-operative and Development

OECD (2010a). *Health care systems: getting more value for money.* Paris, Organisation for Economic Co-operation and Development, (Economics Department Policy Notes).

OECD (2010b). *Value for money in health spending.* Paris, Organisation for Economic Co-operation and Development.

OECD (2011a). *OECD economic surveys: Canada.* Paris, Organisation for Economic Co-operation and Development.

OECD (2011b). *OECD. StatExtracts*. Paris, Organisation for Economic Co-operation and Development (http://stats.oecd.org/Inadex.aspx?DataSetCode=SHA, accessed 25 April 2011).

O'Reilly P (2000). *Health care practitioners: an Ontario case study in policy making.* Toronto: University of Toronto Press.

O'Reilly P (2001). The federal/provincial/territorial health conference system. In: Adams D, ed. *Federalism, democracy and health policy in Canada*. Montreal, McGill-Queen's University Press.

Ostry A (2006). *Change and continuity in Canada's health care system*. Ottawa, CHA Press.

Ouellet R (2004). The effects of international trade agreements and options for upcoming negotiations. In: Marchildon GP, McIntosh T, Forest PG, eds. *The fiscal sustainability of health care in Canada*. Toronto, University of Toronto Press:403–422.

Paris V, Docteur E (2006). *Pharmaceutical pricing and reimbursement policies in Canada.* Paris, (Health Working Paper), Organisation for Economic Co-operation and Development.

Pederson AE, Hack TF (2011). The British Columbia patient navigation model: a critical analysis. *Oncology Nursing Forum*, 38(2):200–206.

PHAC (2008). *Health equity through intersectoral action: an analysis of 18 country case studies*. Ottawa, Public Health Agency of Canada and World Health Organization.

PHAC (2011). *Organized breast cancer screening programs in Canada: report on program performance in 2005 and 2006*. Ottawa, Public Health Agency of Canada.

PHAC & CIHI (2011). *Obesity in Canada*. Ottawa, Public Health Agency of Canada and the Canadian Institute for Health Information.

Philippon DJ, Braithwaite J (2008). Health system organization and governance in Canada and Australia: a comparison of historical developments, recent policy changes and future implications. *Healthcare Policy*, 4(1):e168–e186.

Phillips K (2009). *Catastrophic drug coverage in Canada*. Ottawa, Parliamentary Information and Research Services, Library of Parliament.

Pomey MP, et al. (2007). Public/private partnerships for prescription drug coverage: policy formulation and outcomes in Quebec's universal drug insurance program, with comparisons to the medicare Prescription Drug program. *Milbank Quarterly*, 85(3):469–498.

Pottie K, et al. (2008). Language, proficiency, gender and self-reported health. *Canadian Journal of Public Health*, 99(6):505–510.

Prichard JR (1990). *Liability and compensation in health care*. Toronto, University of Toronto Press.

Quality End-of-Life Care Coalition of Canada (2008). *Hospice palliative home care in Canada: a progress report*. Ottawa, Quality End-of-Life Care Coalition of Canada.

Reid, GJ, et al. (2009). Access to family physicians in southwestern Ontario. *Healthcare Policy*, 5(2):e187–e206.

Requejo F (2010). Federalism and democracy: the case of minority nations: a federalist deficit. In: Burgess M, Gagnon A, eds. *Federal democracies*. London, Routledge:275–298.

Rock G (2000). Changes in the Canadian blood system: the Krever Inquiry, Canadian Blood Services and Héma-Québec. *Transfusion Science*, 22(1):29–37.

Roemer R, Taylor A, Lariviere J (2005). Origins of the WHO Framework Convention on Tobacco Control. *American Journal of Public Health*, 95(6):936–938.

Rogowski W (2007). Current impact of gene technology on healthcare: a map of economic assessments. *Health Policy*, 80(2):340–357.

Romanow RJ (2002). *Building on values: the future of health care in Canada*. Saskatoon, Commission on the Future of Health Care in Canada.

Romanow RJ, Marchildon GP (2003). Psychological services and the future of health care in Canada. *Canadian Psychology*, 44(3):283–298.

Roos N, Mustard CA (1997). Variation in health and health care use by socioeconomic status in Winnipeg, Canada: does the system work well? Yes and no. *Milbank Quarterly*, 75(1):89–111.

Ruggeri J, Watson B (2008). *Federal fiscal abundance and interregional redistribution*. Ottawa, Caledon Institute for Social Policy.

Runnels V, Labonte K, Packer C (2011). Reflections on the ethics of recruiting foreign-trained human resources for health. *Human Resources for Health* 9(2) (http://www.human-resources-health.com/contet/9/1/2, accessed 25 September 2012).

Schoen C, et al. (2009). A survey of primary care physicians in eleven countries, 2009: perspectives on care, costs, and experiences. *Health Affairs*, 28(6):w1171–w1183.

Schoen C, Osborn R, Squires D (2010). How health insurance design affects access to care and costs, by income, in eleven countries. *Health Affairs*, 29(12):w2323–w2334.

Schoen C, Osborn R, Squires D, et al. (2011). New 2011 survey of patients with complex care needs in 11 countries finds that care is often poorly coordinated. *Health Affairs*, online first, 9 November (doi: 10.1377/hithaff.2011.10923).

Sealy P, Whitehead PC (2004). Forty years of deinstitutionalization of psychiatric services in Canada: an empirical assessment. *Canadian Journal of Psychiatry*, 49(4):249–257.

Senate of Canada (2002). *The health of Canadians – the federal role. Final report on the state of the health care system in Canada,* Volume 6. Ottawa, Standing Senate Committee on Social Affairs, Science and Technology.

Senate of Canada (2006). *Out of the shadows at last: transforming mental health, mental illness and addiction services in Canada*. Ottawa, Standing Senate Committee on Social Affairs, Science and Technology.

Senate of Canada (2010). *Raising the bar: a roadmap for the future of palliative care in Canada*. Ottawa, Senate of Canada.

Senate of Canada (2012). *Time for transformative change: a review of the 2004 Health Accord*. Ottawa, Standing Senate Committee on Social Affairs, Science and Technology, Senate of Canada.

Sharma S, Xia C, Roach C, et al. (2010). Assessing dietary intake in a population undergoing a rapid transition in diet and lifestyle: the Arctic Inuit in Nunavut, Canada. *British Journal of Nutrition*, 103:749–759.

Shrybman S (2007). P3 hospitals and the principles of medicare. In: Campbell B, Marchildon GP, eds. *Medicare: facts, myths, problems and promise*. Toronto, Lorimer:197–211.

Siddiqi A, Zuberi D, Nguyen QC (2009). The role of health insurance in explaining immigrant versus non-immigrant disparities in access to health care: comparing the United States to Canada. *Social Science & Medicine*, 69(10):1452–1459.

Simach L (2009). *Health literacy and immigrant populations*. Ottawa, Public Health Agency of Canada (policy brief).

Sims-Gould J, Martin-Matthews A (2010). We share the care: family caregivers' experiences of their older relative receiving home support services. *Health and Social Care in the Community*, 18(4):415–423.

Sinclair D, Rochon M, Leatt P (2005). *Riding the third rail: the story of Ontario's Health Services Restructuring Commission, 1996–2000.* Montreal, Institute for Research on Public Policy.

Smith M (2002). *Patient's bill of rights: a comparative overview.* Ottawa, Library of Parliament, Parliamentary Research Branch.

Smith MJ, Simpson JE (2003). Alternative practices and products: a survival guide. *Health Policy Research Bulletin (Health Canada)*, 7:3–5.

Stabile M, Laporte A, Coyte PC (2006). Household responses to public home care programs. *Journal of Health Economics*, 25(4):674–701.

Stabile M, Ward C (2006). The effects of delisting publicly funded health-care services. In: Beach CM et al. *Health services restructuring in Canada: new evidence and new directions*, Montreal, McGill-Queen's University Press:83–109.

Ståhl T, et al., eds. (2006). *Health in all policies: prospects and potentials.* Helsinki, Ministry of Social Affairs and Health and European Observatory on Health Systems and Policies.

Statistics Canada (2006). *2006 census of population.* Ottawa: Statistics Canada.

Statistics Canada (2008). *Canada's ethnocultural mosaic, 2006 census.* Ottawa, Statistics Canada.

Statistics Canada (2009). *Table 052–0005: projected population, by projection scenario, sex and age group as of July 1, Canada, provinces and territories, annual (persons).* Ottawa: Statistics Canada.

Statistics Canada (2011). *2011 census of population.* Ottawa, Statistics Canada.

Statistics Canada (2012). *Table 202–0705 for income inequality (after-tax Gini coefficient.* Ottawa, Statistics Canada.

Steele LS, et al. (2007). Educational level, income level and mental health service use in Canada: associations and policy implications. *Healthcare Policy*, 3(1):96–106.

Sutherland JM, et al. (2011). British Columbia hospitals: examination and assessment of payment reforms (B-CHeaPR). *BMC Health Services Research* 2011, 11(50): http://biomedcentral.com/1472-6963/11/150.

Sutherland JM (2011a). *Hospital payment mechanisms: an overview and options for Canada.* Ottawa, Canadian Health Services Research Foundation.

Sutherland R (2011b). *False positives: private profit in Canada's medical laboratories.* Halifax, Fernwood Publishing.

Syme A, Bruce A (2009). Hospice and palliative care. What unites us? What divides us? *Journal of Hospice and Palliative Nursing*, 11(1):19–24.

Tarride J, et al. (2008). Economic evaluations conducted by Canadian health technology assessment agencies: where do we stand? *International Journal of Technology Assessment in Health Care*, 24(4):437–444.

Taylor MG (1987). *Health insurance and Canadian public policy: the seven decisions that created the Canadian healthcare systems,* 2nd edn. Montreal, McGill-Queen's University Press.

Tempier R, et al. (2009). Mental disorders and mental health care in Canada and Australia: comparative and epidemiological findings. *Social Psychiatry and Psychiatric Epidemiology*, 44(1):63–72.

Touati N, Pomey MP (2009). Accreditation at a crossroads: are we on the right track? *Health Policy*, 90(2–3):156–165.

Tully P, Saint-Pierre E (1997). Downsizing Canada's hospitals, 1986/87 to 1994/95. *Statistics Canada Health Reports*, 8(4):33–39.

Tuohy CH (2002). The costs of constraint and prospects for health care reform in Canada. *Health Affairs*, 21(3):32–46.

Tuohy CH (2009). Single-payer, multiple systems: the scopes and limits of subnational variation under a federal health policy framework. *Journal of Health Politics, Policy and Law* 34(4):453–496.

Tzountzouris JP, Gilbert JH (2009). Role of educational institutions in identifying and responding to emerging health human resource needs. *Healthcare Papers*, 9(2):6–19.

UNDP (2010). *Human development report 2010. The real wealth of nations: pathways to human development*. New York, United Nations Development Programme.

UNDP (2011). *Human development report 2011*. New York, United Nations Development Programme.

Urowitz S, et al. (2008). Is Canada ready for patient accessible electronic health records? A national scan. *BMC Medical Informatics and Decision Making*, 8: 33 (http://www.biomedcentral.com/1472-6947/8/33, accessed 25 September 2012).

Van Doorslaer E, Masseria C (2004). *Income-related inequality in the use of medical care in 21 OECD countries*. Paris, Organisation for Economic Co-operation and Development.

Wackinshaw E (2011). Patient navigators becoming the norm in Canada. *Canadian Medical Association Journal*, 183(15):E1109–E1110.

Wadden N (2005). Breast cancer screening in Canada: a review. *Canadian Association of Radiologists Journal,* 56(5):271–275.

Waldrum JB, Herring DA, Young TK (2006). *Aboriginal health in Canada: historical, cultural and epidemiological perspectives*, 2nd edn. Toronto, University of Toronto Press.

Wallace BB, MacEntee MI (2011). Access to dental care for low-income adults: perceptions of affordability, availability and acceptability. *Journal of Community Health*, 37(1):32–39..

Watanabe M, Comeau M, Buske L (2008). Analysis of international migration patterns affecting physician supply in Canada. *Healthcare Policy*, 3(4):e129–e138.

Watts RL (2008). *Comparing federal systems*. 3rd edn. Kingston, McGill-Queen's University Press for the Institute of Intergovernmental Relations.

Welsh S, et al. (2004). Moving forward? Complementary and alternative practitioners seeking self-regulation. *Sociology of Health and Illness*, 26(2):216–241.

WHO (2003). *Framework convention on tobacco control*. Geneva, World Health Organization.

WHO (2007). *Neonatal and perinatal mortality: country, regional and global estimates 2004*. Geneva, World Health Organization.

WHO (2010). *World health statistics 2010*. Geneva, World Health Organization.

WHO (2011). *Mortality Database*. Geneva, World Health Organization. (http://who.int/healthinfo/morttables/en/, accessed 18 April 2011).

WHO (2011a). *Global health observatory data repository*. Geneva, World Health Organization. (http://apps.who.int/ghodata, accessed 25 April 2011).

Widger K, et al. (2007). Pediatric patients receiving palliative care in Canada. *Archives of Pediatrics & Adolescent Medicine*, 161(6):597–602.

Wilkins K (2006). Government-subsidized home care. *Statistics Canada Health Reports*, 17(4):39–42.

Wilkins K, Shields M (2009). Colorectal cancer screening in Canada – 2008. *Statistics Canada Health Reports*, 20(3):1–11.

Williams AM, et al. (2010). Tracking the evolution of hospice palliative care in Canada: a comparative case study analysis of seven provinces. *BMC Health Services Research*, 10:147.

Williams AM, et al. (2011). Canada's compassionate care benefit: is it an adequate public health response to addressing the issue of caregiver burden in end-of-life care? *BMC Public Health*, 11:335.

Wilson DM, et al. (2008). The rapidly changing location of death in Canada, 1994–2004. *Social Science & Medicine*, 68(10):1752–1758.

Wiktorowicz M, et al. (2003). Nonprofit groups and health policy in Ontario: assessing strategies and influence in a changing environment. In: Brock KL, ed. *Delicate dances: public policy and the nonprofit sector*. Kingston, McGill-Queen's University Press for School of Policy Studies, Queen's University:171–219.

Wolfson S (1997). Use of paraprofessionals: the Saskatchewan Dental Plan. In: Glor E, ed. *Policy innovation in the Saskatchewan public sector*. Toronto, Captus Press.

World Bank (2011). Data. Washington DC, World Bank. (http://data.worldbank.org/, accessed 21 April 2011).

Wranik D (2008). Health human resource planning in Canada: a typology and its application. *Health Policy*, 86(1):27–41.

Wright M, et al. (2008). Mapping levels of palliative care development: a global view. *Journal of Pain and Symptom Management*, 35(5):469–485.

Young TK, Chatwood S (2011). Health care in the north: what Canada can learn from its circumpolar neighbours. *Canadian Medical Association Journal*, 183(2):209–214.

9.2 Useful web sites

9.2.1 Federal government

Canada Health Act: http://www.laws-lois.justice.gc.ca/eng/acts/C-6/

Health Canada: http://www.hc-sc.gc.ca

Mental Health Commission of Canada: http://www.mentalhealthcommission.ca/

Patented Medicine Prices Review Board: http://www.pmprb-cepmb.gc.ca/

Public Health Agency of Canada: http://www.phac-aspc.gc.ca/

Statistics Canada: http://www.statcan.gc.ca

9.2.2 Provincial and territorial health ministries

Alberta: Alberta Health and Wellness: http://www.health.alberta.ca/

British Columbia: Ministry of Health: http://www.gov.bc.ca/health/

Manitoba: Manitoba Health: http://www.gov.mb.ca/health/

New Brunswick: Department of Health: http://www.gnb.ca/0051/index-e.asp

Newfoundland and Labrador: Department of Health and Community Services: http://www.health.gov.nl.ca/health/

Northwest Territories: Department of Health and Social Services: http://www.hlthss.gov.nt.ca/

Nova Scotia: Department of Health and Wellness: http://www.gov.ns.ca/DHW/

Nunavut: Department of Health and Social Services: http://www.hss.gov.nu.ca/en/

Ontario: Ministry of Health and Long-Term Care: http://www.health.gov.on.ca/

Prince Edward Island: Department of Health and Wellness: http://www.gov.pe.ca/health/

Quebec: Ministère de la Santé et Services sociaux: http://www.msss.gouv.qc.ca

Saskatchewan: Ministry of Health: http://www.health.gov.sk.ca/

Yukon: Department of Health and Social Services: http://www.hss.gov.yk.ca/

9.2.3 Selected intergovernmental organizations

Canada Health Infoway: https://www.infoway-inforoute.ca/

Canadian Agency for Drugs and Technologies in Health: http://www.cadth.ca/

Canadian Blood Services: http://www.blood.ca

Canadian Institute for Health Information: http://www.cihi.ca

Canadian Intergovernmental Conference Secretariat: http://www.scics.gc.ca

Canadian Partnership Against Cancer Corporation: http://www.partnershipagainstcancer.ca/

Canadian Patient Safety Institute: http://www.patientsafetyinstitute.ca/

Council of the Federation: http://www.councilofthefederation.ca/

Health Council of Canada: http://www.healthcouncilcanada.ca/

Pan-Canadian Public Health Network: http://www.phn-rsp.ca/

9.2.4 Provincial health agencies of note

Alberta: Health Quality Council: http://www.health.alberta.ca/services/hqca.html

British Columbia: Patient Safety and Quality Council: http://www.bcpsqc.ca

New Brunswick: Health Council: http://www.nbhc.ca

Nova Scotia: Health Care Safety and Quality: http://www.gov.ns.ca/health/health_care_safety

Ontario: Cancer Care Ontario: http://www.cancercare.on.ca

Ontario: Cardiac Care Network of Ontario: http://www.ccn.on.ca

Ontario: Health Quality Ontario: http://www.ohqc.ca

Ontario: Hospital Association: http://www.oha.com

Ontario: Institute for Clinical Evaluative Sciences: http://www.ices.on.ca

Quebec: Héma-Québec: http://www.hema-quebec.qc.ca/

Quebec: La Régie de l'assurance maladie du Quebec: http://www.ramq.gouv.qc.ca/

Quebec: L'Institut national d'excellence en santé et en services sociaux: http://www.inesss.qc.ca/

Saskatchewan: Health Quality Council: http://www.hqc.sk.ca

9.2.5 Selected pan-Canadian health provider organizations

Association of Faculties of Medicine of Canada: http://www.afmc.ca/

Canadian Association of Medical Physicists: http://www.medphys.ca/

Canadian Association of Medical Radiation Technologists: http://www.camrt.ca

Canadian Association of Midwives: http://www.canadianmidwives.org/

Canadian Association of Naturopathic Doctors: http://www.naturopathicassoc.ca

Canadian Association of Occupational Therapists: http://www.caot.ca

Canadian Association of Optometrists: http://opto.ca/

Canadian Association of Physician Assistants: http://capa-acam.ca

Canadian Association of Social Workers: http://www.casw-acts.ca/

Canadian Association of Speech-Language Pathologists and Audiologists: http://www.caslpa.ca/

Canadian Chiropractic Association: http://www.chiropracticcanada.ca/

Canadian Dental Association: http://www.cda-adc.ca/

Canadian Dental Hygienists Association: http://www.cdha.ca/

Canadian Health Information Management Association: https://www.echima.ca/

Canadian Institute of Public Health Inspectors: http://www.ciphi.ca/

Canadian Medical Association: http://www.cma.ca

Canadian Nurses Association: http://www.cna-aiic.ca/

Canadian Osteopathic Association: http://www.osteopathic.ca/

Canadian Pharmacists Association: http://www.pharmacists.ca

Canadian Physiotherapy Association: http://www.physiotherapy.ca

Canadian Psychological Association: http://www.cpa.ca/

Canadian Public Health Association: http://www.cpha.ca/

Canadian Society for Medical Laboratory Science: http://www.csmls.org/

Canadian Society of Respiratory Therapists: http://www.csrt.com/

Collège des médicins du Québec: http://www.cmq.org

College of Family Physicians of Canada: http://www.cfpc.ca

Dietitians of Canada: http://www.dietitians.ca

Homeopathic Medical Association of Canada: http://www.hmac.ca/

Natural Health Practitioners of Canada: http://www.nhpcanada.org/

Registered Psychiatric Nurses of Canada: http://www.rpnc.ca

Royal College of Dentists of Canada: http://www.rcdc.ca

Royal College of Physicians and Surgeons of Canada: http://www.royalcollege.ca/

9.2.6 National non-profit-making organizations

Alzheimer Society of Canada: http://www.alzheimer.ca

Arthritis Society: http://www.arthritis.ca

Association of Canadian Academic Healthcare Organizations: http://www.acaho.org

Association of Workers' Compensation Boards of Canada: http://www.awcbc.org

Asthma Society of Canada: http://www.asthma.ca

Autism Canada Foundation: www.autismcanada.org

Canada's Research-based Pharmaceuticals Companies: https://www.canadapharma.org/

Canadian AIDS Society: http://www.cdnaids.ca

Canadian Association for Community Care: http://www.cacc-acssc.com

Canadian Association of Retired Persons: http://www.50plus.com

Canadian Breast Cancer Network: http://www.cbcn.ca

Canadian Cancer Society: http://www.cancer.ca

Canadian Council on Health Services Accreditation: http://www.accreditation.ca/

Canadian Cystic Fibrosis Foundation: http://www.cysticfibrosis.ca/

Canadian Diabetes Association: http://www.diabetes.ca

Canadian Down Syndrome Society: http://www.cdss.ca

Canadian Generic Pharmaceutical Association: http://www.canadiangenerics.ca/

Canadian Health Coalition: http://www.healthcoalition.ca

Canadian Healthcare Association: http://www.cha.ca

Canadian Hemophilia Society: http://www.hemophilia.ca

Canadian Homecare Association: http://www.cdnhomecare.ca

Canadian Hospice Palliative Care Association: http://www.chpca.net

Canadian Life and Health Insurance Association: http://www.clhia.ca

Canadian Liver Foundation: http://www.liver.ca/

Canadian Lung Association: http://www.lung.ca

Canadian Medical Foundation: http://www.medicalfoundation.ca

Canadian Mental Health Association: http://www.cmha.ca

Canadian National Institute for the Blind: http://www.cnib.ca

Canadian Organization for Rare Disorders: http://www.raredisorders.ca/

Canadian Psychiatric Research Foundation: http://healthymindscanada.ca/

Canadian Society for Medical Laboratory Science: http://www.csmls.org

Canadian Transplant Society: http://cantransplant.ca/

Canadian Women's Health Network: http://www.cwhn.ca

Cystic Fibrosis Canada: http://www.cysticfibrosis.ca

Epilepsy Canada: http://www.epilepsy.ca

Health Charities Coalition of Canada: http://www.healthcharities.ca

Heart and Stroke Foundation of Canada: http://www.heartandstroke.ca

Huntington Society of Canada: http://www.huntingtonsociety.ca/

Kidney Foundation of Canada: http://www.kidney.ca

Medical Council of Canada: http://www.mcc.ca

Multiple Sclerosis Society of Canada: http://www.mssociety.ca

Muscular Dystrophy Association of Canada: http://muscle.ca

National Network for Mental Health: http://www.nnmh.ca

Osteoporosis Society of Canada: http://www.osteoporosis.ca

Parkinson Society Canada: http://www.parkinson.ca

Prostate Cancer Canada Network: http://www.prostatecancer.ca

9.2.7 Selected health services and policy research (including funding) organizations

Atlantic Health Promotion Research Centre: http://www.ahprc.dal.ca

Canadian Association for Health Services and Policy Research: http://www.cahspr.ca

Canadian Consortium for Health Promotion Research (University of Toronto): http://www.utoronto.ca/chp/CCHPR

Canadian Health Services Research Foundation: http://www.chsrf.ca/

Canadian Institute of Child Health: http://www.cich.ca

Canadian Institutes of Health Research: http://www.cihr-irsc.gc.ca

Centre for Addiction and Mental Health: http://www.camh.net

Centre for Evidence-based Medicine: http://ktclearinghouse.ca/cebm/

Centre for Health Economics and Policy Analysis (McMaster University): http://www.chepa.org

Centre for Health Evidence: http://www.cche.net

Centre for Health Promotion (University of Toronto): http://www.utoronto.ca/chp

Centre for Health Promotion Studies (University of Alberta): http://www.chps.ualberta.ca

Centre for Health Services and Policy Research (Queen's University): http://chspr.queensu.ca

Centre for Health Services and Policy Research (University of British Columbia): http://www.chspr.ubc.ca

Centre for Rural and Northern Health Research (Laurentian University): http://cranhr.laurentian.ca

Centres of Excellence for Women's Health: http://www.cewh-cesf.ca

Coalition for Research in Women's Health: http://www.crwh.org

Genome Canada: http://www.genomecanada.ca

Health Law Institute (University of Alberta): http://www.law.ualberta.ca/centres/hli/

Institute of Health Economics: http://www.ihe.ca

Institute for Work and Health: http://www.iwh.on.ca

Manitoba Centre for Health Policy (University of Manitoba): http://www.umanitoba.ca/centres/mchp

National Alliance of Provincial Health Research Organizations: http://www.nbhrf.com/national-alliance-provincial-health-research-organizations :

- Alberta Innovates: Health Solutions: http://www.ahfmr.ab.ca/
- Fonds de la recherche en santé du Québec: http://www.frsq.gouv.qc.ca/fr/index.shtml
- Manitoba Health Research Council: http://www.mhrc.mb.ca/
- Michael Smith Foundation for Health Research (BC): http://www.msfhr.org/
- New Brunswick Health Research Foundation: http://www.nbhrf.com/
- Newfoundland and Labrador Centre for Applied Health Research: http://www.nlcahr.mun.ca/
- Nova Scotia Health Research Foundation: http://www.nshrf.ca/
- Saskatchewan Health Research Foundation: http://www.shrf.ca/

National Network on Environments and Women's Health:
http://www.nnewh.org/

Population Health Research Institute (McMaster University):
http://www.phri.ca

Population Health Research Unit (Dalhousie University):
http://www.phru.dal.ca/

9.3 Selected laws on health and health care in Canada

9.3.1 Federal laws

Access to Information Act, RSC 1985, c C-49

Assisted Human Reproduction Act, SC 2004, c 2

Canada Consumer Product Safety Act, SC 2010, c 21

Canada Health Act, RSC 1985, c C-6

Canada Marine Act, SC 1998, c 10

Canadian Environmental Protection Act, 1999, SC 1999, c 33

Canadian Food Inspection Agency Act, SC 1997, c 6

Controlled Drugs and Substances Act, SC 1996, c 19

Department of Health Act, SC 1996, c 8

Emergencies Act, RSC 1985, c 22

Federal–Provincial Fiscal Arrangements Act, RSC 1985, c F-8

Food and Drugs Act, RSC 1985, c F-27

Human Pathogens and Toxins Act, SC 2009, c 24

Immigration and Refugee Protection Act, SC 2001, c 27

Indian Act, RSC 1985, c I-5

Nuclear Safety and Control Act, SC 1997, c 9

Patent Act, RSC 1985, c P-4

Personal Information Protection and Electronic Documents Act, SC 2000, c 5

Privacy Act, RSC 1985, c P-21

Public Health Agency of Canada Act, SC 2006, c 5

Quarantine Act, SC 2005, c 20

Radiation Emitting Devices Act, RSC 1985, c R-1

Tobacco Act, SC 1997, c 13

Veterans Insurance Act, RSC 1970, c V-3

9.3.2 Provincial and territorial laws pertaining to medicare

Alberta
Hospitals Act, RSA 2000, c H-12
Alberta Health Care Insurance Act, RSA 2000, c A-20

British Columbia
Hospital Insurance Act, RSBC 1996, c 204
Medical Protection Act, RSBC 1996, c 286

Manitoba
Health Services Insurance Act, CCSM, c H-35

New Brunswick
Hospital Services Act, RSNB 1973, c H-9
Medical Services Payment Act, RSNB 1973, c M-7

Newfoundland
Hospital Insurance Agreement Act, RSNL 1990, c H-7
Medical Care Insurance Act, SNL 1999, c M-5.1

Northwest Territories
Hospital Insurance and Health and Social Services Administration Act, RSNWT 1988, c M-8
Medical Care Act, RSNWT 1988, c M-8

Nova Scotia
Health Services and Insurance Act, RS 1989, c 197

Nunavut (adopted existing laws from Northwest Territories when created in 1999)
Hospital Insurance and Health and Social Services Administration Act, RSNWT 1988, c M-8
Medical Care Act, RSNWT 1988, c M-8

Ontario
Health Insurance Act, RRO 1990, c H-6

Prince Edward Island
Hospital and Diagnostic Services Insurance Act, RSPEI 1988, c H-8
Health Services Payment Act, RSPEI 1988, c H-2

Quebec
Hospital Insurance Act, RSQ, c A-28
Health Insurance Act, RSQ, c A-29

Saskatchewan
Saskatchewan Medical Care Insurance Act, RSS 1978, c S-29

Yukon
Hospital Insurance Services Act, RSY 2002, c 112
Health Care Insurance Plan Act, RSY 2002, c 107

9.4 HiT methodology and production process

HiTs are produced by country experts in collaboration with the Observatory's research directors and staff. They are based on a template that, revised periodically, provides detailed guidelines and specific questions, definitions, suggestions for data sources and examples needed to compile reviews. While the template offers a comprehensive set of questions, it is intended to be used in a flexible way to allow authors and editors to adapt it to their particular national context. The most recent template is available online at: http://www.euro.who.int/en/home/projects/observatory/publications/health-system-profiles-hits/hit-template-2010.

Authors draw on multiple data sources for the compilation of HiTs, ranging from national statistics, national and regional policy documents to published literature. Furthermore, international data sources may be incorporated, such as those of the OECD and the World Bank. The OECD Health Data contain over 1200 indicators for the 34 OECD countries. Data are drawn from information collected by national statistical bureaux and health ministries. The World Bank provides World Development Indicators, which also rely on official sources.

In addition to the information and data provided by the country experts, the Observatory supplies quantitative data in the form of a set of standard comparative figures for each country, drawing on the European Health for All database. The Health for All database contains more than 600 indicators defined by the WHO Regional Office for Europe for the purpose of monitoring Health in All Policies in Europe. It is updated for distribution twice a year from various sources, relying largely upon official figures provided by governments, as well as health statistics collected by the technical units of the WHO Regional Office for Europe. The standard Health for All data have been officially approved by national governments. With its summer 2007 edition, the Health for All database started to take account of the enlarged EU of 27 Member States.

HiT authors are encouraged to discuss the data in the text in detail, including the standard figures prepared by the Observatory staff, especially if there are concerns about discrepancies between the data available from different sources.

A typical HiT consists of nine chapters.

1. Introduction: outlines the broader context of the health system, including geography and sociodemography, economic and political context, and population health.
2. Organization and governance: provides an overview of how the health system in the country is organized, governed, planned and regulated, as well as the historical background of the system; outlines the main actors and their decision-making powers; and describes the level of patient empowerment in the areas of information, choice, rights, complaints procedures, public participation and cross-border health care.
3. Financing: provides information on the level of expenditure and the distribution of health spending across different service areas, sources of revenue, how resources are pooled and allocated, who is covered, what benefits are covered, the extent of user charges and other out-of-pocket payments, voluntary health insurance and how providers are paid.
4. Physical and human resources: deals with the planning and distribution of capital stock and investments, infrastructure and medical equipment; the context in which IT systems operate; and human resource input into the health system, including information on workforce trends, professional mobility, training and career paths.
5. Provision of services: concentrates on the organization and delivery of services and patient flows, addressing public health, primary care, secondary and tertiary care, day care, emergency care, pharmaceutical care, rehabilitation, long-term care, services for informal carers, palliative care, mental health care, dental care, complementary and alternative medicine, and health services for specific populations.

6. Principal health reforms: reviews reforms, policies and organizational changes; and provides an overview of future developments.
7. Assessment of the health system: provides an assessment based on the stated objectives of the health system, financial protection and equity in financing; user experience and equity of access to health care; health outcomes, health service outcomes and quality of care; health system efficiency; and transparency and accountability.
8. Conclusions: identifies key findings, highlights the lessons learned from health system changes; and summarizes remaining challenges and future prospects.
9. Appendices: includes references, useful web sites and legislation.

The quality of HiTs is of real importance since they inform policy-making and meta-analysis. HiTs are the subject of wide consultation throughout the writing and editing process, which involves multiple iterations. They are then subject to the following.

- A rigorous review process (see the following section).
- There are further efforts to ensure quality while the report is finalized that focus on copy-editing and proofreading.
- HiTs are disseminated (hard copies, electronic publication, translations and launches). The editor supports the authors throughout the production process and in close consultation with the authors ensures that all stages of the process are taken forward as effectively as possible.

One of the authors is also a member of the Observatory staff team and they are responsible for supporting the other authors throughout the writing and production process. They consult closely with each other to ensure that all stages of the process are as effective as possible and that HiTs meet the series standard and can support both national decision-making and comparisons across countries.

9.5 The review process

This consists of three stages. Initially the text of the HiT is checked, reviewed and approved by the series editors of the European Observatory. It is then sent for review to two independent academic experts, and their comments and amendments are incorporated into the text, and modifications are made accordingly. The text is then submitted to the relevant ministry of health, or appropriate authority, and policy-makers within those bodies are restricted to checking for factual errors within the HiT.

9.6 About the author

Gregory Marchildon holds a Canada Research Chair (Tier 1) at the Johnson–Shoyama Graduate School of Public Policy at the University of Regina in Canada. After receiving his PhD at the London School of Economics, he taught at Johns Hopkins University's School of Advanced International Studies. He then became a senior civil servant in Canada and the Executive Director of a Royal Commission on the future of health care in Canada. A fellow in the Canadian Academy of Health Sciences, his current research interests include comparative health systems with a focus on circumpolar countries, decentralization and policy history.

Index